METABOLISM DIET FOR BEGINNERS

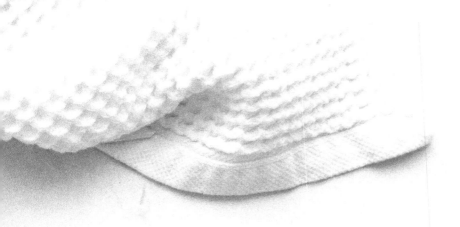

METABOLISM DIET FOR BEGINNERS

2-Week Meal Plan and Exercises to Kick-Start Weight Loss

Megan Johnson McCullough

Photography by Annie Martin

ROCKRIDGE
PRESS

Interior and Cover Designer: Julie Schrader
Art Producer: Meg Baggott
Editor: Rebecca Markley
Production Editor: Nora Milman
Photography © 2021 Annie Martin. Food styling by Nadine Page Beauchamp.
Illustrations © 2020-21 Charlie Layton
Author photo courtesy of Kathy Magerkurth

ISBN: Print 978-1-64876-619-0 | eBook 978-1-64876-118-8
R0

This plan is dedicated to anyone who seeks to improve, better themselves, and aim for being the best version of themselves.

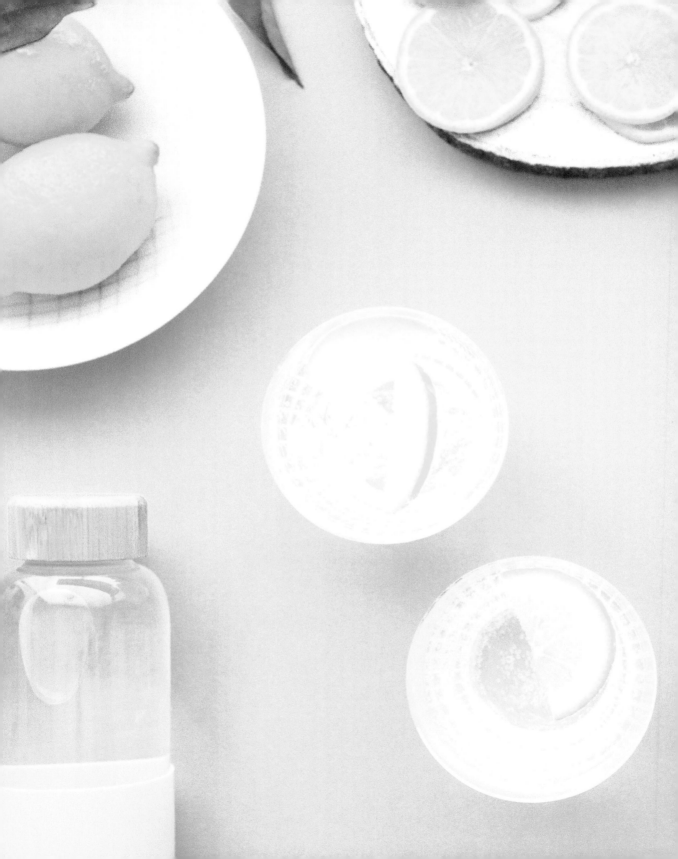

CONTENTS

INTRODUCTION

I'm Megan Johnson McCullough and let me start by saying how incredibly thankful I am to share this metabolism plan with you. As the owner of Every BODY's Fit fitness studio in Oceanside, California, a professional natural bodybuilder, an NASM Master Trainer, published author, and candidate for a doctorate in health and human performance, my mission is to help every BODY become the best version of themselves.

My relationship with diet and exercise has been an exhausting game of overeating and trying to erase the guilt with exercise. As an athlete my whole life and as a college basketball player, I've always eaten healthily. No fast food, no soda, and rare treats, but I also never skip a meal or leave anything on my plate. As I've aged and become more educated, my metabolism is now at peak performance because I've changed my mindset and played to my strengths.

A plan like this is exactly what I turned to when I was nearly 50 pounds overweight. At that time, I knew that almonds were a healthy snack, but not the entire bag of almonds. Portion distortion ruled my life after knee surgery and being homesick in college. Even after becoming educated in nutrition and until I became a natural bodybuilder, I didn't know what one serving size meant. Ranking second in the world in natural bodybuilding meant no longer letting food control me.

Your body will reward you when you care for it and nourish it with the healthy attention it is begging for. Food is the fuel you are putting in your tank, and junk won't make your engine work efficiently. Exercise is medicine and movement is healing, mentally and physically. Where you are today and where you will be days from now—and beyond—will prove to you that you are worth this journey, and each step will lead to an improved quality of life. Nothing changes if nothing changes, so let's make a change . . . your metabolism is ready to work with you.

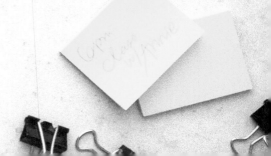

PART I

THE FOUNDATION

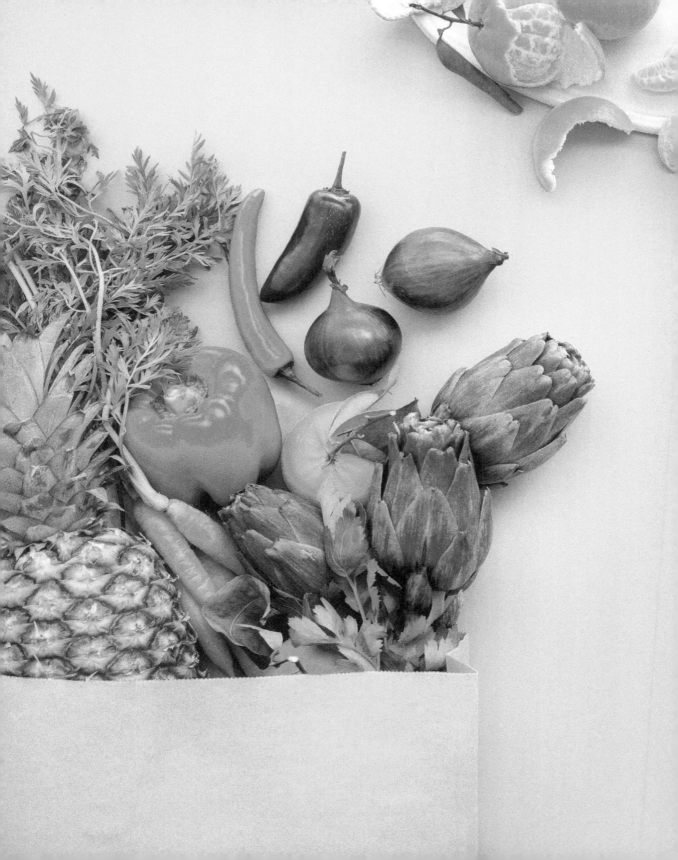

CHAPTER 1

What You Need to Know

When it comes to weight loss, metabolism can be the telltale factor associated with the success of any form of diet or exercise. Your success for this plan is understanding that here today, you are starting a new, scientifically based weight loss journey tailored to your body's metabolic functioning. You will experience a change in what you see in the mirror and what you feel inside when you stay honest with your efforts and decide to commit to this new lifestyle change of improvement. Make the promise today to put yourself in the driver's seat of your metabolism.

Know the Approach

Your metabolism converts food to energy and is the maintenance system necessary to perform bodily functions. Ever heard someone point the finger at their "slow" metabolism for not being able to lose weight? The bigger picture is what you are eating and what activities you are doing.

Kick-Start Your Best Self into Action

This is the beginning of a new chapter of getting your metabolism to work for you, rather than against you. Changing behaviors can be uncomfortable at first, but start with just two weeks on the agenda and let the rest happen later. Be in the moment. Think of it as one day at a time, not 14.

Fresh Start

Do not let past experiences haunt you or deter you from treating yourself to this plan. If something didn't work before or you tend to stop and start or have tried everything in the past, be resilient. Your body will thank you for the opportunity ahead and your commitment to bettering yourself via your metabolism.

Think Intrinsic

Not every measure of progress is numerical or bound to what the scale reads. Other measures of progress include improved sleep, better-fitting clothes, and higher energy levels. Maybe you can even walk up the stairs without losing your breath. Your quality of life is headed in the right direction.

Plan Ahead

Prep meals, shop for groceries, and set your alarm. Keeping a schedule establishes routine. Once routine is developed, just like your metabolism, you become trained to care for yourself. Cooking and exercise become prioritized and part of your agenda. Over time, fewer distractions persist, and you look forward to this plan.

There is no perfect start date. There will always be birthdays, holidays, work projects, and social ties. Your metabolism exists regardless. Do not procrastinate any longer. This plan is a lifestyle change that is sustainable, so if you have a bad day, get right back on track the next day. Setbacks happen and when they do, pause, then pivot yourself in the right direction. Don't quit. You can do this.

Know Your Metabolism

Your metabolism is the process in which your body converts what you eat and drink each day into energy. Straightforward math: The calories in the food you eat plus the calories in the drinks you consume plus oxygen equals (and releases) the energy your body needs to function.

What Is Your Metabolism and How Does It Function?

After we eat and drink, the digestive system goes to work by firing up enzymes (proteins that cause chemical reactions) to turn fat into fatty acids, convert carbohydrates into simple sugars (called glucose), and break down proteins into amino acids. Glucose is the body's main fuel in the gas tank. These compounds (fat, carbohydrates, protein) get absorbed in our blood and are delivered to the cells. The body stores or releases the compounds, resulting in a two-part process:

1. Anabolism is the construction zone, responsible for building and storing energy. It helps grow new cells, maintain the health of body tissue, and store energy. This usually takes place right after eating.

2. Catabolism is the action of the cells breaking down and producing energy. This breakdown consists mainly of carbohydrates and fats. Catabolism fuels anabolism by warming our bodies and igniting our muscles to work, which then makes the body move. Anything we don't need becomes waste products that get released and removed through the skin, lungs, kidneys, and intestines.

Hormones are part of our endocrine system, which steers our metabolism and controls the speed. Hormones are also what makes metabolism complicated. There are a few key hormones that act as the dictators. For example, the pancreas decides whether your metabolism is going to act using the anabolic or catabolic process. It is the glucose detector, so after eating, when glucose suddenly rises, the pancreas calls upon insulin, which then signals the anabolic process to start.

Another key hormone to watch out for is called thyroxine. The thyroid gland releases this hormone, which is the culprit for the speed of your metabolism. Now those terms hyper- and hypothyroidism make sense (over and underactive).

The best way we can take care of our metabolism is by fueling our bodies with the right types of calories. Calories are the measurement of how much energy is in a particular food. We either fuel our engine with calories that will burn efficiently or with calories that will be stored for later (fat). This eating plan therefore aligns calories with metabolic functioning for successful weight loss. The amount of calories we should consume should take into consideration our activity level and basal metabolic rate (BMR), which is how many calories our body burns at rest and during daily living activities.

Factors Beyond Your Control

You have probably asked yourself, "What makes my metabolism fast or slow?" Everyone's metabolism is affected by a number of factors. Some can be mitigated but others are difficult to change.

AGE
Resting metabolic rate decreases with age. This is partly due to the decrease in muscle mass as we get older. The more muscle mass the body has, the more fat that is burned. Body fat also tends to accumulate with age. Less energy is expended as the body becomes less active. Glucose tolerance also decreases, which is the body's ability to respond to sugar. Without lifestyle changes, we become more susceptible to type 2 diabetes.

GENETICS
The efficiency of your metabolism can be inherited from your parents. You cannot change your genes. What you are born with can either result in a fast

or slow metabolism. If you were born with thyroid problems, this would influence the speed of your metabolism. Genetics don't influence your weight, but they do play a role in the speed of your metabolism, which then contributes to your body's shape, size, and weight.

HORMONES

The key hormones that affect metabolism include cortisol, thyroid, insulin, and testosterone in men and progesterone in women. Cortisol is the stress regulator, thyroid is the hormonal leader, insulin responds to glucose, and the sex hormones deal with energy and fat storage. When any of these four hormones are imbalanced, metabolism can pay the price. For example, if cortisol levels are high from increased stress, insulin can become more resistant and thyroid production is reduced.

PRESCRIBED MEDICATIONS

Some medications have been found to slow metabolism. These include antidepressants and antipsychotics, medications used for hormone therapy, and some diabetes medications, as well as steroids. Remedies to help with this interaction can be changing the time of day when the medication is taken, changing the dosage, and changing the medication type. Certain high blood pressure medications can also slow metabolism. Not only do some medications slow metabolism, but this can be coupled with increased appetite and difficulty exercising, which in turn can lead to weight gain.

Factors You Can Control

The good news is that there are several factors you can control to help your metabolism. Your success will reflect your ability to take care of these factors, which you CAN do.

WHAT YOU EAT

What foods you choose to serve yourself has either hindered or helped you arrive at your current weight. With this plan, you are being given nutritionally sound recipes that also taste good. Preparing them yourself also puts you in control of what you are consuming. The menu has been selected to help your metabolism, so enjoy this opportunity to be your body's gourmet chef. No more last-minute decisions or emotionally based snacking. It's time to control what goes in.

HOW MUCH YOU MOVE YOUR BODY

Movement is medicine that makes your body feel alive. Being sedentary only shortens the expiration date on your body's joints and muscles. Being active releases positive endorphins and wakes up your entire system by pumping blood to your muscles and letting your heart and lungs come to life. Let standing be the new sitting and let cardio and strength training be part of the daily attention that you give yourself. It's time to burn calories.

HOW MUCH YOU SLEEP

When your body lacks sleep, it doesn't have the chance to clear body fat, which leads to the accumulation of lipids and weight gain. Poor sleep elevates ghrelin, the hunger hormone, making your appetite spike. Simultaneously, leptin, which suppresses appetite, is lowered. The more time we spend awake, the more opportunity we have to take in calories.

Also, rest and recovery are an integral part of this process. In order to sustain this new lifestyle, you want to pace yourself. Burning out only means starting over. Therefore, try to go to sleep at a decent bedtime according to the time you need to wake up in the morning. At minimum, six hours of sleep is needed, but there is no set number for anyone. Listen when your body tells you that it's time to lie down.

YOUR STRESS LEVEL

Life will never be problem-free, but you can control how you react to situations. Expect stumbles and speed bumps, but understand that you can take a deep breath and redirect the course. Make sure that your environment allows you time to yourself. Everyone is given the same 24 hours in a day, so don't worry about what you cannot control. Instead, focus on what you can control and that is starting and sticking to this plan.

YOUR SUPPORT SYSTEM

You don't have to feel isolated or alone for the next 14 days. Share what you are doing with those who will encourage, support, and help you stay accountable. There are people in your life who want to see you do well. Turn to them and let them know you are taking control of your eating and exercise. You might even ask them to join in or you might inspire them to take control for themselves.

STRESS RELIEF

Stress is the body's response to triggers that cause physical or psychological distress. To fight this surge in cortisol, it is important to provide the body with the opportunity to release positive endorphins. This can be done by exercising regularly, keeping a mindset of gratitude by focusing on what you are thankful for, enjoying a good laugh by surrounding yourself with encouraging friends and family, trying yoga to improve the mind-body connection, and making a to-do list that prioritizes your time efficiently. In a world that says "go, go, go," sometimes slowing down will actually help keep your metabolism from slowing.

Know Yourself

The next 14 days are all about YOU taking control of your metabolism and your health. You are being given the action plan, now you must be confident and committed with each step. Be open-minded and receptive to this change. Following this plan is not hard. Everyday life throws many difficult things at you that are much more challenging. Problems will never cease to exist and there will never be a perfect time to start working toward better health. You have accomplished and finished much harder feats in life than this. Cooking your meals and drinking plenty of water is not hard. Accept that your body deserves this change and focus on the short term. Think like a child who wakes up ready for just today, and only today. At the start, you might feel fragile and worried, but these normal feelings will begin to subside as you take control one day at a time.

Know Your "Why"

WHY you chose this plan will be the foundation of your adherence to the next 14 days. Did you have a health scare? Did your doctor recommend that you change your eating habits? Are you trying to get off certain medications?

Are you tired of being tired? Do you want to be more physically capable of performing activities that you once loved or enjoy? Do you want to be a better partner, parent, or grandparent to loved ones? Do you want to fit into your clothes again? Do you feel depressed or discouraged by your body image? Be passionate about your WHY. The HOW is right in front of you, but the WHY will serve as your motivation and inspiration to draw upon through this process and to remind you of your progress, where you started, and how far you have come. Your WHY is your starting line; now you are ready to go.

Know Your "How"

Think about your current habits and behaviors. What do you prioritize in your life and what are your commitments? Consider the routines and timeline of your days. Certain changes will be required for success. You may need to rearrange your thought processes and gear them toward this program and the to-do list related to accomplishing your metabolic goal. Prepare yourself to be able to plan your meals, incorporate exercise, get enough rest, and shift your attitude to believing that you will follow through with the goals for each of the next 14 days. Bring this written plan to action.

Know Your "When"

The perfect two weeks might never exist, but do start this plan at an optimal time when you can diligently focus on your body and health. This doesn't mean procrastinating until the stars align, but it means looking at the near future and deciding the 14 days that will best set yourself up for success. If you are a stress eater or emotional eater and have upcoming events such as holidays that could trigger these tendencies, steer clear of these times to start. You must also have availability for exercise. Ultimately, you will make the time for what is important to you.

Know Your Kitchen

Now it's time to put those kitchen appliances to work. Your mind and body are ready to rumble, and the kitchen is ready to use some electricity. Get your kitchen equipped and let it become a space for your health's improvement. Create an environment that matches your intentions.

Clean Out Your Pantry

Like it or not, the junk has to go. Clean out your kitchen because it is time for clean eating. Eliminate what could taunt you and make the items that you crave or turn to for mindless eating disappear. You have a new grocery list to make space for.

FOODS NOT ALLOWED ON THE PLAN

- ☐ Alcohol
- ☐ Bagels
- ☐ Battered foods
- ☐ Candy bars or candy of any type
- ☐ Canned soups
- ☐ Chips
- ☐ Coffee specialty drinks
- ☐ Croissants and danishes
- ☐ Dips for chips
- ☐ Donuts
- ☐ Energy drinks
- ☐ Fast food
- ☐ Fried foods
- ☐ Frozen dinners
- ☐ Frozen pizzas
- ☐ Granola bars and fruit-filled bars
- ☐ Gum with sugar
- ☐ Hot dogs, bratwurst, and corn dogs
- ☐ Jelly and jams
- ☐ Lemonade
- ☐ Milkshakes
- ☐ Prepackaged burritos
- ☐ Prepackaged donuts, cookies, muffins, biscuits, and cakes
- ☐ Prepackaged ketchup, barbecue sauce, and salad dressings

- ☐ Prepackaged oatmeal
- ☐ Prepackaged ramen noodles, macaroni and cheese, and crackers
- ☐ Prepackaged smoothies
- ☐ Prepackaged specialty breads such as banana or blueberry
- ☐ Soda
- ☐ Sports drinks
- ☐ Sugary cereals
- ☐ Trail mixes and pretzels
- ☐ White bread products
- ☐ Yogurt with pre-added fruit or flavors

Stock-Up Staples

What you can enjoy are high-quality foods that serve a purpose in your body. Better yet, when you eat right you actually get to eat more because you aren't eating high-calorie, high-fat options. Some staples to stock up on include nondairy milk, nuts, brown rice, whole-wheat pastas and breads, fruits and vegetables, and lean proteins like chicken breast, ground turkey, and fish such as tilapia, salmon, and cod.

FOODS TO ENJOY

These grab-and-go options will help satisfy cravings and hunger (two or fewer options per day):

- ☐ ¼ cup (24) almonds, lightly salted
- ☐ 1 or 2 dill pickle slices
- ☐ 1 or 2 hard-boiled eggs
- ☐ ½ piece whole-wheat toast with 2 ounces avocado
- ☐ 1 sugar-free Jell-O cup
- ☐ 4 ounces sweet potato with cinnamon
- ☐ Celery sticks with 1 piece string cheese
- ☐ 2 slices turkey breast with 1 piece string cheese
- ☐ Cucumber, whole or sliced
- ☐ 1 cup nonfat plain Greek yogurt or 1 cup nonfat cottage cheese

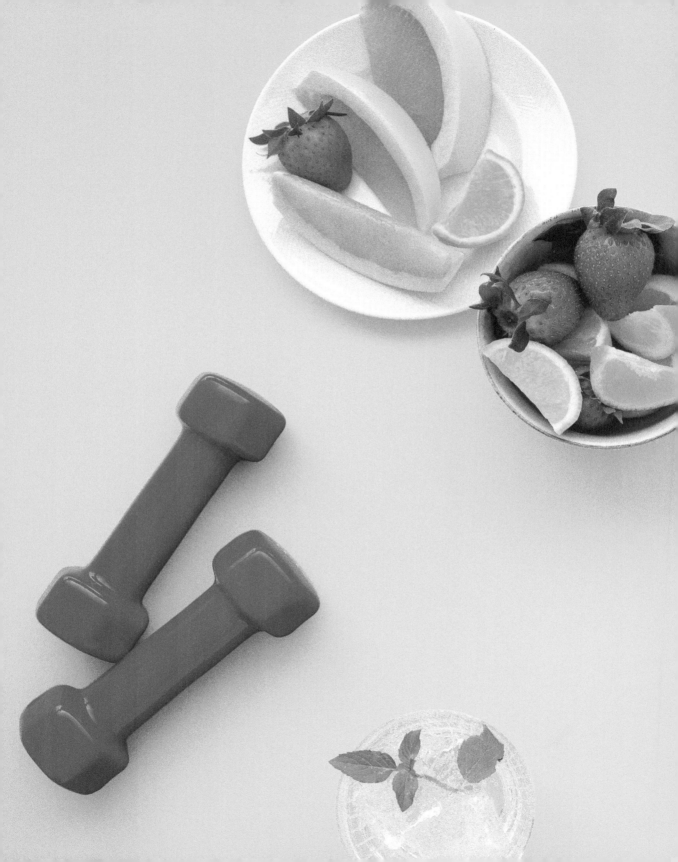

CHAPTER 2

Steps to Success

You are being presented with working information, which means that you must put these guidelines into action. Each day of these two weeks is a day spent learning about how to improve yourself. In doing so, each day you will feel accomplished and proud of every indication of progress. No one but you can do this for you, so be ready to work hard, be your body's leader, and once you decide in your mind that you are going to do this plan, your body has no choice but to follow. Are you ready to work for what you want?

Make Time to Exercise

Exercise is movement and activity that is both mentally and physically rewarding. Regular exercise will boost your health, and it can help ward off health conditions such as type 2 diabetes, heart disease, high blood pressure, depression, anxiety, and arthritis, and, of course, it can aid the functioning of your metabolism. It can also help you fall asleep faster. Exercise during this program, and for the rest of your life, will put more pep in your step by increasing your energy level.

Making time for exercise and having the motivation to do so doesn't require any fancy equipment or extravagant workout. Consistency is the key, so you might try incorporating exercise at the start of your day, at the end of your day, or in the middle to break up your day. You can also break up your exercise into small increments throughout the day. Any amount of exercise is better than none at all. Your body is a machine that wants to burn calories, so when you use your energy systems to exercise, the blood starts pumping, and the body appreciates the opportunity to move. Remember that your metabolism is the conversion of food to energy, so the more energy you expend, the more calories you burn.

Cardio

Cardio is any type of exercise that raises your heart rate. This involves the aerobic system, which helps your oxygen function more efficiently, and the cardiovascular system, which includes the heart and lungs. Common examples include biking, walking, swimming, or dancing. There are a number of benefits and reasons to do cardio, including boosting your mood through the release of positive endorphins, burning calories, strengthening your heart and lungs, achieving better sleep, and warding off diabetes, high blood pressure, and heart disease. Feeling a little short of breath or breathing harder tells you that the heart is working, and those calories are burning.

Strength

Strength training, also known as resistance training, involves contracting the muscles while resisting a force. This can be done with bodyweight, free weights, or machines in a pushing or pulling manner. The best part about strength training is that it boosts your metabolism because your body will burn more calories at rest when you incorporate this type of exercise. Simply put, the more lean muscle you have, the more calories you burn (even when watching TV). Strength training also improves bone density, which helps ward off osteopenia and osteoporosis. Don't fear the weights or worry that you will become bulky if that is not your goal. You will get stronger and tone your body, but you train for the results you want to see. Therefore, if bulking is your goal, you would lift much heavier weights and change your diet accordingly for building muscle mass. Here, we are focused on the afterburn effect that strength training has on your body.

The Exercises

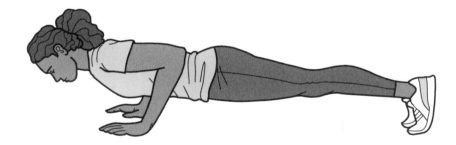

PUSH-UPS

Start with your feet and hands shoulder-width apart, holding yourself up in a tabletop position. Look 6 feet in front of you on the floor. Keep the neck neutral and slowly descend toward the floor until your elbows are even with your ears. Once in alignment, push yourself back up to the starting position. **Modification:** This exercise can be performed on the knees or even standing and pushing yourself away from a wall.

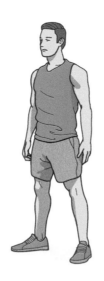
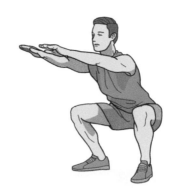

SQUATS

Stand with your feet shoulder-width apart, toes pointed forward. Slowly lower your body toward the floor (imagine sitting down in a chair) until your knees and quadriceps (thighs) are in a 90-degree bent position. Keep your chest up and eyes looking forward, then stand back up, pushing through your heels and squeezing your glutes (bottom) as you return to the starting-standing position. **Modification:** If your knees hurt, you can widen your stance and slightly point the toes outward.

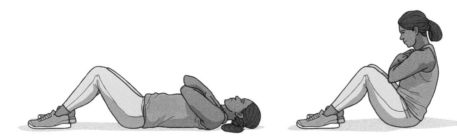

SIT-UPS

Start on the floor, lying with your knees bent and feet shoulder-width apart. Place your hands across your chest. Take a deep breath and peel your spine off the floor, bringing your chest toward your knees. **Modification:** If you are unable to fully sit up, just lift your shoulder blades off the floor (considered a "crunch"). You can also use your arms for momentum to lift your spine off the floor.

REVERSE LUNGES

Stand with your feet shoulder-width apart, toes pointed forward. Step 1 foot back and lower your body into a 90-degree stance with the back foot now on the ball of your toes. After the position is reached, step the leg that is in back to the starting position. Alternate and step the other foot back, repeating the sequence with proper form. **Modification:** It is okay if your range of motion is less than 90 degrees. Just go as far as you can.

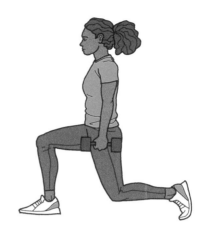

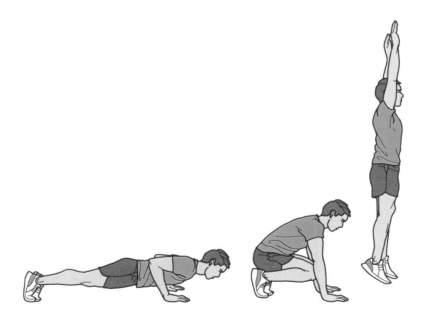

BURPEES

Start in the tabletop plank position (think of the starting position of a push-up on your toes). Jump both feet in toward your chest, then stand your body upright. For an added calorie burn, take a small jump as soon as you stand up. Then jump or step your feet back to the starting tabletop position to repeat the activity. **Modification:** Rather than jumping your feet, you can step them in and out. You can use an elevated surface such as a chair for assistance.

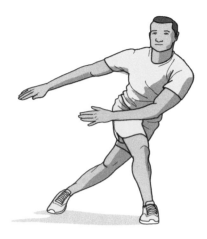
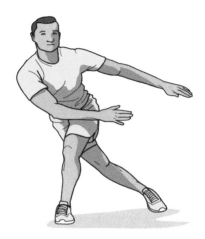

ICE SKATERS

Start in a standing position and step your right leg back and across your left leg. Simultaneously reach across your right arms toward your left ankle. In a fast motion, leap side to side, crossing the leg behind and reaching the arm down and across to increase heart rate for this cardio exercise. For an extra challenge, reach and touch the opposite toe during this motion. Be mindful of your lower back when reaching downward. **Modification:** Rather than leaning over to reach for your ankle, you can reach for your shin or knee for a lesser range of motion to accommodate for low back pain.

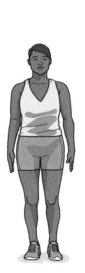
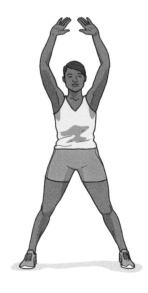

JUMPING JACKS

Start in a standing position and jump both your feet outside your shoulders while also raising your arms over your head, bringing the hands close together. Repeat this motion, jumping the feet in and out while raising the arms up and down. **Modification:** For a lower impact move, step-tap the feet outward while raising the arms to replace the jumping movement. This cardio exercise will elevate your heart rate efficiently.

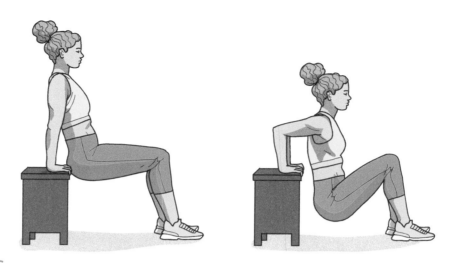

DIPS

Using a chair, bench, or any elevated surface, stand facing away from the equipment. Place your palms with your fingers pointed toward your body onto the surface, lowering your body until your knees are bent in a 90-degree position and your feet are shoulder-width apart. Lower yourself down, keeping the elbows inward to a range that brings your palms close to your rib cage. Then straighten the arms as you raise yourself back to the start. **Modification:** Instead of lowering your body 90 degrees, just take your bottom on and off the platform you are using while holding yourself up. Try to move your body forward off the platform then back to the platform with your palms on the surface.

CHAIR STANDS

Place a chair on a stable surface and sit down, making sure your feet are parallel, shoulder width apart, and that your toes are pointed forward. Pushing through your heels, stand up. Squeeze your glutes (bottom) as you straighten and stand back up. Continue to sit and stand, elevating the heart rate and targeting the lower body. Weights can be held for added resistance to strengthen the legs.

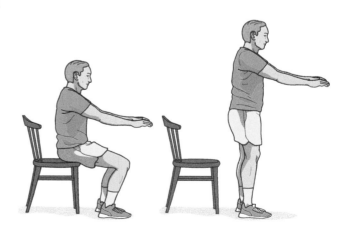

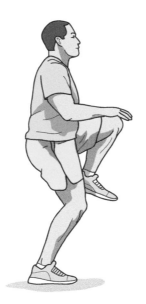 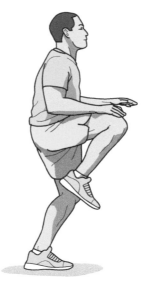

HIGH KNEES

Start with your feet shoulder-width apart and place your palms, facedown, in front of your body near your hips. Tap your right knee to your right palm, then your left knee to your left palm. Repeat this motion, alternating quickly. You can do this at a marching pace or, for an extra cardio burst, try to have one foot off the ground at all times in a more hopping motion (you are trying not to have both feet on the ground at the same time).

The Plans

The following mini plans are developed for persons who do not regularly exercise or have little experience doing so. These bodyweight exercises build a foundation for cardio and strength training that can be performed anywhere. The initial two weeks of exercise will focus on building endurance and stamina. Remember to listen to your body and lessen your intensity or stop when you feel lightheaded, dizzy, or overheated. Take a moment to drink water. Modifications are available for most exercises. Keep in mind that no workout is a bad workout, so keep moving and do what you can as best as you can within your body's ability.

MINI PLAN 1

You'll need a stopwatch for timed intervals. Begin by doing Jumping Jacks for 45 seconds, then Chair Stands for 45 seconds, then repeat these two exercises 8 to 10 times each. Repeat this same pattern with Ice Skaters for 45 seconds and Reverse Lunges for 45 seconds, completing each exercise 8 to 10 times. Finish by holding a plank for 30 seconds to 1 minute. Incorporate a 20- to 30-minute walk that elevates your heart rate.

MINI PLAN 2

This is a 10x5 workout. Perform 10 Squats, 10 Sit-Ups, 10 Burpees, and 10 Dips a total of 5 sets each. If you have access to a staircase, walk up and down for 10 minutes OR if you do not have stairs, do an interval walk at a quick pace for 2 minutes then a normal walking pace for 1 minute. Repeat this for 18 to 24 minutes.

MINI PLAN 3

Perform 3 to 5 sets of the following exercises for 12 to 20 repetitions: Push-Ups, Squats, Jumping Jacks, and Dips. Next, time yourself for 30 seconds to 1 minute of High Knees followed by 12 to 20 Sit-Ups for 3 to 5 sets of each. The number of repetitions and sets will depend on your endurance and if you hold extra hand weights or not. You can track your progress and increase reps and sets over time.

MINI PLAN 4

Perform 3 to 5 sets of 40 Ice Skaters (each step is one rep) and 20 to 40 alternating Reverse Lunges. Next, perform 3 to 5 sets of 40 High Knees (each leg is one rep) and 12 to 20 Chair Stands. Work at a pace that elevates your heart rate. Take a 30-second rest in between sets (if needed). Finish by holding a 30-second to 1-minute long plank.

MINI PLAN 5

Begin by jogging or marching in place for 3 minutes. Then perform 1 minute of Burpees and 1 minute of Sit-Ups. Repeat the 3 minutes of jogging or marching and two exercises for 5 sets. Next, go for a 10- to 15-minute brisk walk or 10 to 15 minutes of walking stairs. Finish with 3 minutes of Chair Stands (just one time). Hold a Plank, timing yourself for as long as you can.

Stay Hydrated

Drinking water to stay hydrated will be extremely important over the next 14 days to help with digestion and exercise recovery. It acts like WD-40 for your joints. I know that some of us don't remember to drink water and some don't really like it, but try to keep a water bottle handy. You can add lemon, cucumber, or mint for good flavor. Keep drinking throughout the day; it can be just a few sips at a time. Don't wait until you are thirsty. Drinking water will help balance sodium and potassium in your body (electrolytes), help with mental focus, and help your cells repair. This is important because you want to stay feeling energized for the entire 14 days. This doesn't mean you have to chug water but be mindful and try to avoid alcohol and caffeine in excess, which do make you feel more dehydrated.

Get Your Zzzzzzzzzz

Sleep is the body's downtime to recharge and recover to prepare for the next day. Lack of sleep can impact your metabolism because imbalances can occur in the body. For example, hormones like cortisol can increase, as well as ghrelin, which then increases your appetite. In turn, leptin (the hormone that regulates appetite) can release in lower amounts, and the body starts to signal that it is hungry. Poor sleep can also lead to poor decision-making as your brain tries to function in a "foggy" and tired state. You can also become more vulnerable to late-night snacking. Not having enough sleep diminishes your energy levels, and your motivation or ability to exercise becomes compromised. This is because many of the body's systems have to rest to help with cellular repair. Without this time, immunity becomes suppressed and you become a "zombie" running on very little steam.

METABOLISM MYTHS

There are many metabolism myths out there, with false claims that you can make your metabolism operate at lightning speed. You must understand that a starvation diet doesn't work, meaning cutting major calories won't make you lose weight faster. Nor does the concept of skipping meals, or thinking that not having breakfast will make you burn off last's night meal faster. Going low-fat or no-fat also doesn't work metabolic magic. Going into saunas and steam rooms won't rev up the speed.

You don't have to excessively cut out caffeine or salt. Having few to no carbs won't work wonders. Spicing up all your entrées and eating peppers to warm up the body to burn more calories isn't necessary, either. Don't envy lean or "skinny" people who appear to be able to eat whatever they want and not gain a pound. They don't have a faster metabolism; in fact, larger people who weigh more actually burn more total calories in a day. There also is not an optimal time of day to exercise when you will burn more calories, or any special meal or drink to have before or after a workout.

If any of these tricks actually worked, there would certainly not be a need for this plan. Let science-based evidence be your guide. Treat your body with quality food and exercise, and the reward will be a well functioning metabolism that burns fat and calories at just the right speed.

Weigh Yourself at the Same Time of Day

If your goal is weight loss, it is important to step on the scale at the same time of day each day. The morning is the optimal time, before you start to consume calories. Wearing the same attire is also necessary for more accurate results. Be sure to weigh yourself on the same scale each day, as scales can be calibrated differently. Keep your scale in a visible place, reminding you of your accountability. After the initial 14 days, you don't have to become scale obsessive. Check in with the scale once or twice a week to keep you honest and on track.

Take Before and After Photos

You see yourself every moment of every day. You are also surrounded by many of the same people each day. Little changes are changes and each change is important. You don't always recognize or "see" these changes day by day as they are taking place. Take a before photo on day 1 and an after photo on day 14. Face forward, on both sides, and turn around. Wear the same attire for all the pictures. You will be able to see it and believe it for yourself. Progress photos remind you of your WHY and keep you inspired to continue.

Keep a Journal

For the next 14 days, write down all that you accomplish each day. This can include what you ate to the details of your mini plans for exercise. Note your reps and sets and any weights used. Describe how you felt. Jot down your emotions. This journal will be a great reference to recall recipes you loved, triggers that you want to avoid in the future, and your physical improvement from cardio and resistance training. This is your report card for accountability. Taking a moment to evaluate your day can help steer you in the right direction moving forward or make changes for the next day.

Set Realistic Expectations

Be realistic: Your weight did not accumulate overnight, nor will it disappear overnight. What you put into this program is what you will get of it. You don't have to be perfect, but you do have to be realistic about your expectations. Food is a constant in our lives that we can't just give up and instantly fix. We have to eat to live, so now the choice is deciding that we will no longer live to eat. Train your mind to relate food to nourishment and fuel for the body, not a pleasure-seeking and taste-bud–based occurrence.

About the Plan

Everything over the next two weeks has been organized and strategically planned for you. Be confident with the tools you are being provided, including shopping lists, meal plans, and exercise plans. Look forward to healthy weight loss, sustainable lifestyle changes, and liking what you see in the mirror. Watch your endurance and strength progress with exercise. Watch your clothes start to fit better. Watch the people around you notice your increased energy and better mood. Enjoy cooking recipes that are structured to benefit your body with nourishment. Keep in mind that there are labels for allergens and substitutions available. You will learn about the connection between your mind and body, and even after these 14 days feel encouraged to continue taking care of yourself. When you feel good, you become a better person to yourself and those you love. Health is wealth, and your improved metabolism is worth millions.

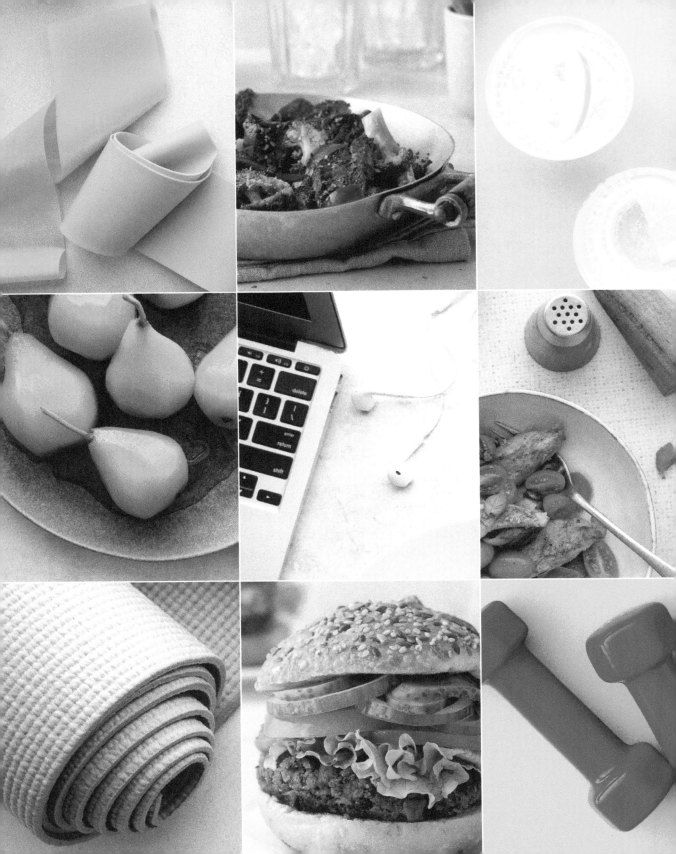

CHAPTER 3

The 2-Week Plan

Week 1

I t's time to get this plan going—you can do this. You will realize after these next 14 days that you are a metabolism champion for taking charge of your health. After that, don't look back because that is not where you are headed. With the tools you learn, you will be stronger, mentally and physically, because this lifestyle change will become a positive mindset you won't want to let go of. Whatever you think you should have, could have, or would have been before, it doesn't matter. Here today, and from now on, YOU ARE A LEADER OF SELF-CARE.

SHOPPING LIST

PANTRY / SHELF-STABLE

- ☐ Almond butter
- ☐ Apricots, dried
- ☐ Black pepper, ground
- ☐ Brown rice
- ☐ Chia seeds
- ☐ Chili powder
- ☐ Chipotle chili powder
- ☐ Cinnamon, ground
- ☐ Coconut sugar or similar substitute for granulated sugar
- ☐ Cranberries, dried
- ☐ Cumin, ground
- ☐ Dark chocolate chips
- ☐ Dijon mustard
- ☐ Fish sauce
- ☐ Garlic powder
- ☐ Hamburger buns, whole-wheat, 4
- ☐ Italian herbs, dried
- ☐ Maple syrup, pure
- ☐ Oats, old-fashioned
- ☐ Oil, olive, extra-virgin
- ☐ Oregano, dried
- ☐ Pita rounds, whole-wheat, 4
- ☐ Quinoa
- ☐ Red pepper flakes
- ☐ Sea salt
- ☐ Soy sauce, low-sodium
- ☐ Spaghetti noodles, whole-wheat, 3 ounces
- ☐ Thyme, dried
- ☐ Tortillas, whole-wheat, 4 (7-inch)
- ☐ Vinegar, balsamic
- ☐ Vinegar, red wine
- ☐ Walnuts, pieces

CANNED AND BOTTLED

- ☐ Artichoke hearts, water-packed, 2 (15-ounce) cans
- ☐ Black beans, 1 (15-ounce) can
- ☐ Black olives, sliced, 1 (2-ounce) can
- ☐ Chicken broth, low-sodium, 6 cups
- ☐ Dill pickles, 1 jar
- ☐ Roasted red peppers, 1 (12-ounce) jar
- ☐ Tomatoes with garlic and basil, chopped, 1 (15-ounce) can
- ☐ Tomatoes, crushed, 1 (14-ounce) can

PRODUCE

- ☐ Apple, banana, or orange, 1
- ☐ Avocado, 1
- ☐ Baby spinach, 7 cups
- ☐ Basil leaves, 10
- ☐ Bell peppers, any color, 5
- ☐ Bell peppers, red, 3
- ☐ Carrots, 2
- ☐ Cherry tomatoes, 1 pint
- ☐ Cilantro, 1 bunch
- ☐ Cremini mushrooms, 8 ounces
- ☐ Dill, 1 bunch
- ☐ Edamame, 1 cup
- ☐ Garlic, 1 head
- ☐ Grapes, 1 cup
- ☐ Jalapeño pepper, 1
- ☐ Kale, 2 cups
- ☐ Lemons, 3
- ☐ Onions, red, 3
- ☐ Onions, yellow, 4
- ☐ Shallot, 1
- ☐ Strawberries, 1 pint
- ☐ Summer squash (zucchini, pattypan, yellow), medium, 4
- ☐ Sweet potatoes, 6

DAIRY AND EGGS / REFRIGERATED

- ☐ Eggs, large, 16

- ☐ Greek yogurt, nonfat, plain, 3½ cups

- ☐ Jell-O cups, sugar-free, 1 package

- ☐ Milk, skim, 2½ cups

- ☐ Parmesan cheese, shredded, 2 ounces

- ☐ String cheese sticks, 1 package

PROTEINS

- ☐ Chicken breast, boneless, skinless, 8 ounces

- ☐ Chicken breast, boneless, skinless, cooked, 2 cups

- ☐ Ground beef, extra-lean, 1 pound

- ☐ Halibut, 4 (4-ounce) fillets

- ☐ Tofu, extra-firm, 8 ounces

- ☐ Turkey bacon, 4 slices

- ☐ Turkey breast, deli sliced, 12 ounces

WEEK 1 MEAL PLAN

	MEAL	SELECTION
DAY 1	Breakfast	Cranberry-Cinnamon Overnight Oats (page 52)
	Snack 1	Baked Sweet Potato Chips (page 152)
	Lunch	Turkey, Cranberry, and Spinach Pinwheels (page 85)
	Snack 2	1 sugar-free Jell-O cup
	Dinner	Veggie and Brown Rice–Stuffed Bell Peppers (page 104)

	MEAL	SELECTION
DAY 2	Breakfast	Leftover Cranberry-Cinnamon Overnight Oats
	Snack 1	1 cup Greek yogurt or 1 cup nonfat cottage cheese
	Lunch	Leftover Turkey, Cranberry, and Spinach Pinwheels
	Snack 2	1 or 2 dill pickles
	Dinner	Herbed Halibut and Summer Squash in Parchment (page 110)

	MEAL	SELECTION
DAY 3	Breakfast	Kale, Red Pepper, and Turkey Bacon Egg Cups (page 64)
	Snack 1	Leftover Baked Sweet Potato Chips
	Lunch	Black Bean–Stuffed Sweet Potatoes (page 94)
	Snack 2	Almond Butter Chocolate Chip Cookies (page 161)
	Dinner	Leftover Veggie and Brown Rice–Stuffed Bell Peppers

continued >

	MEAL	SELECTION
DAY 4	Breakfast	Leftover Kale, Red Pepper, and Turkey Bacon Egg Cups
	Snack 1	1 sugar-free Jell-O cup
	Lunch	Chicken Noodle Soup (page 78)
	Snack 2	1 cup Greek yogurt or 1 cup nonfat cottage cheese
	Dinner	Italian-Inspired Chopped Salad (page 74)

	MEAL	SELECTION
DAY 5	Breakfast	Quinoa, Oat, and Apricot Breakfast Bars (page 55)
	Snack 1	1 to 2 hard-boiled eggs
	Lunch	Leftover Black Bean–Stuffed Sweet Potatoes
	Snack 2	Leftover Almond Butter Chocolate Chip Cookies
	Dinner	Easy Pub-Style Burgers (page 137)

	MEAL	SELECTION
DAY 6	Breakfast	Southwest Tofu Scramble (page 58)
	Snack 1	2 slices turkey breast with 1 piece string cheese
	Lunch	Leftover Chicken Noodle Soup
	Snack 2	Leftover Almond Butter Chocolate Chip Cookies
	Dinner	Leftover Easy Pub-Style Burgers

	MEAL	SELECTION
DAY 7	Breakfast	Leftover Quinoa, Oat, and Apricot Breakfast Bars
	Snack 1	¼ cup (24) almonds, lightly salted
	Lunch	Veggie Pita Pizzas (page 99)
	Snack 2	1 piece string cheese and celery sticks
	Dinner	Strawberry and Spinach Salad (page 70)

REAL LIFE SKILL: BUILDING A HEALTHY MEAL ON THE GO

Life keeps going while you're on this plan, which means eating out is very possible. Don't worry, it won't derail your results. You don't have to live in total isolation; in fact, you shouldn't. Keep in mind the tools and tips that you have learned and make this plan part of your life, so that you can sustain the changes. As soon as you feel deprived and restricted, it is likely you will let your accomplishments go, one by one. Instead, consider what your plate should look like when you go out. Stick to lean meats that include 2 to 5 ounces of protein (or about the size of a deck of cards), such as poultry, fish, tofu, or pork. Choose whole-wheat or whole-grain starches and starchy vegetables like potatoes and yams that are about the size of a baseball, or 1 cup. You can have one baseball and a half of green leafy vegetables, which is about 3 cups raw or 1½ cups cooked. Select fruits that are about the size of a baseball, or about 1 cup. If possible, look at the menu ahead of time. Ask for sauces on the side. The two-bite rule comes in handy when pressured to eat foods you are trying to avoid: Take two bites and move on. You were polite and reasonable. Don't become antisocial just because food is social. Be confident that you are fully equipped with the tools to prioritize your health, regardless of the environment.

Week 2

Congratulations on all that you have accomplished! Time flies when you are headed on the right path. Doesn't it feel good to feel good? Think about the chef you have become, the exerciser you are now, and the leader by example you represent to others. You took control and you took charge. This change for better has motivated you to keep getting better. Your body wants to give you a 5-star review and huge thank-you. Be proud of every moment of progress because you deserve recognition. Here's to never seeing that starting number on the scale seven days ago, ever again.

SHOPPING LIST

*Be sure to check your kitchen for items like spices that you have already used and purchased. If you have leftovers from Week 1, you can substitute them in the menu accordingly.

PANTRY / SHELF-STABLE

- ☐ Baking soda
- ☐ Black pepper, ground
- ☐ Bread, whole-grain, 1 loaf
- ☐ Capers
- ☐ Chili powder
- ☐ Cinnamon
- ☐ Coriander, ground
- ☐ Cumin, ground
- ☐ Dijon mustard
- ☐ Fish sauce
- ☐ Flour, whole-wheat
- ☐ Garlic powder
- ☐ Honey
- ☐ Maple syrup
- ☐ Mayonnaise

- ☐ Oats, old-fashioned
- ☐ Oil, avocado
- ☐ Oil, olive, extra-virgin
- ☐ Oregano
- ☐ Pumpkin pie spice
- ☐ Quinoa
- ☐ Red pepper flakes
- ☐ Rice cakes, 1 package
- ☐ Sea salt
- ☐ Smoked paprika
- ☐ Sriracha (optional)
- ☐ Thyme
- ☐ Vanilla extract
- ☐ Vinegar, red wine

CANNED AND BOTTLED

- ☐ Almond milk or nondairy milk of choice, plain, unsweetened, ¾ cup
- ☐ Chicken broth, low-sodium, ½ cup
- ☐ Kidney beans, low-sodium, 2 (15-ounce) cans
- ☐ Lentils, 2 (15-ounce) cans
- ☐ Pumpkin puree, 1 (15-ounce) can
- ☐ Roasted red peppers, jarred, ¼ cup
- ☐ Tomatoes, crushed, 1 (14.5-ounce) can
- ☐ Tomatoes, crushed, 2 (28-ounce) cans
- ☐ Tuna, water-packed, 2 (5-ounce) cans
- ☐ Water chestnuts, sliced, 1 (8-ounce) can

PRODUCE

- ☐ Apple, banana, or orange, 1
- ☐ Avocado, 1
- ☐ Baby carrots, 10 ounces
- ☐ Baby spinach, 2 cups
- ☐ Bananas, ripe, 3
- ☐ Basil leaves, 10
- ☐ Bell pepper, green, 1
- ☐ Brussels sprouts, 10 ounces
- ☐ Celery, 2 stalks
- ☐ Cherry tomatoes, 10
- ☐ Cilantro, 1 bunch
- ☐ Cucumber, 1
- ☐ Dill, 1 bunch
- ☐ Fennel bulb, 1
- ☐ Garlic (1 head)
- ☐ Ginger, 1 (3-inch) knob
- ☐ Green cabbage, shredded, 1 cup
- ☐ Jalapeño pepper, 1
- ☐ Lemons, 3
- ☐ Lime, 1
- ☐ Mangos, 2
- ☐ Mixed berries, fresh or frozen (strawberries, blueberries, blackberries, raspberries), 4 cups
- ☐ Onion, red, 1
- ☐ Onions, yellow, 2

- ☐ Scallions, 1 bunch

- ☐ Shallots, 7

- ☐ Shiitake mushrooms, sliced, 8 ounces

- ☐ Sweet potato, 4 ounces

DAIRY AND EGGS

- ☐ Eggs, large, 2 dozen

- ☐ Greek yogurt, plain, nonfat, 1½ cups

- ☐ Milk, skim, 4 cups

- ☐ Parmesan cheese, shredded, 2 tablespoons (optional)

PROTEINS

- ☐ Chicken thighs, bone-in, 4

- ☐ Ground beef, extra-lean, 1 pound

- ☐ Tilapia, 4 (4-ounce) fillets

- ☐ Turkey, 4 (3-ounce) cutlets

WEEK 2 MEAL PLAN

	MEAL	SELECTION
DAY 8	Breakfast	Pumpkin Spice Smoothie (page 47)
	Snack 1	Roasted Red Pepper Deviled Eggs (page 155)
	Lunch	Vegan Chili (page 90)
	Snack 2	1 or 2 dill pickles
	Dinner	Ginger-Cilantro Meatballs (page 136)

	MEAL	SELECTION
DAY 9	Breakfast	Leftover Pumpkin Spice Smoothie
	Snack 1	1 piece string cheese and cucumbers
	Lunch	Tilapia with Mango Salsa (page 112)
	Snack 2	Leftover Roasted Red Pepper Deviled Eggs
	Dinner	Roasted Chicken Thighs and Root Vegetables (page 119)

	MEAL	SELECTION
DAY 10	Breakfast	Open-Faced Avocado Toast Breakfast Sandwich (page 57)
	Snack 1	1 apple
	Lunch	Leftover Tilapia with Mango Salsa
	Snack 2	Creamy Mixed Berry Freezer Pop (page 163)
	Dinner	Leftover Ginger-Cilantro Meatballs

	MEAL	SELECTION
DAY 11	Breakfast	Mushroom and Spinach Frittata (page 60)
	Snack 1	1 sugar-free Jell-O cup
	Lunch	Leftover Vegan Chili
	Snack 2	1 or 2 dill pickles
	Dinner	Leftover Roasted Chicken Thighs and Root Vegetables

	MEAL	SELECTION	
DAY 12	Breakfast	Whole-Grain Banana Muffins (page 56)	
	Snack 1	Celery sticks and 1 piece string cheese	
	Lunch	Dilled Tuna Salad Sandwich (page 83)	
	Snack 2	1 medium sweet potato with cinnamon	
	Dinner	Mediterranean Spiced Lentils and Quinoa (page 96)	

	MEAL	SELECTION	
DAY 13	Breakfast	Leftover Mushroom and Spinach Frittata	
	Snack 1	1 apple	
	Lunch	Turkey Piccata (page 116)	
	Snack 2	1 sugar-free Jell-O cup	
	Dinner	Leftover Mediterranean Spiced Lentils and Quinoa	

	MEAL	SELECTION	
DAY 14	Breakfast	Leftover Whole-Grain Banana Muffins	
	Snack 1	1 or 2 rice cakes	
	Lunch	Leftover Dilled Tuna Salad Sandwich	
	Snack 2	Leftover Creamy Mixed Berry Freezer Pop	
	Dinner	Leftover Turkey Piccata	

REAL LIFE SKILL: MAINTENANCE MODE

Continuing this plan will offer lifelong health. By staying on this healthy path, you are mitigating potential health risks and adding to your quality of life. If you can do it for 14 days, maintain this state of mind one day at a time moving forward. Remember, one day at a time.

How to Maintain and Continue Your Weight Loss

In order to keep and maintain the results you have achieved, it will be important to stay active and continue to plan your meals in advance. Make sure your kitchen is stocked with the good foods you can have and the go-to snacks that keep you in line. You will also need to prepare the majority of your meals. Don't revert back to convenience and the drive-thru. If you had the time before, you have the time now, too. Be smart about desserts and indulgences. You don't have to deprive yourself entirely or have an all-or-nothing attitude, but be realistic about your strengths and weaknesses. Staying consistent is the key. Whatever kept you in line before, continue to do the same things now. That might be weighing yourself once a week to keep yourself accountable. Don't beat yourself up if you have slipups. Vacations, parties, and holidays will always exist.

What If I Didn't Lose Weight?

The scale is not your only indication of the success and progress of this plan. Never let the scale define you. Circumference measurements also reveal the reshaping of your body. Consider your waistline. Do your pants fit better? Do your tops feel looser? Your activity level has also increased. Can you do more than when you started any of the exercises? Do you not get out of breath as easily? Has your quality of sleep improved? You might have more energy in the day and feel in a better mood more often than not. You also do not know what improved internally. Have your blood pressure and cholesterol checked to see if they have become lower. If you are still concerned, you can always seek the advice of your doctor. Have a comprehensive blood panel performed to check your thyroid and hormones, making sure they are balanced. **Do not give up and remember your WHY.**

Next Steps

Your daily schedule has changed to prioritize your health. Keep this schedule. Continue to use your shopping list, prepare your meals at home, stick to portion control, and exercise three to five days or more per week. Your body has noticed your hard work, so keep your mind motivated to keep going. Set new goals with realistic expectations to strive for. Think of a reward to earn and work for, such as a vacation or gift you have always wanted to treat yourself to. Express to those you spend your time with that you intend to continue this plan. It is possible they see what you have accomplished and want to take part. Whether you know it or not, you have inspired others. Keep your kitchen and personal environment optimal for your continued success. Remember to tell yourself you are worth this. **Remember your WHY because now you know HOW.**

PART II

THE RECIPES

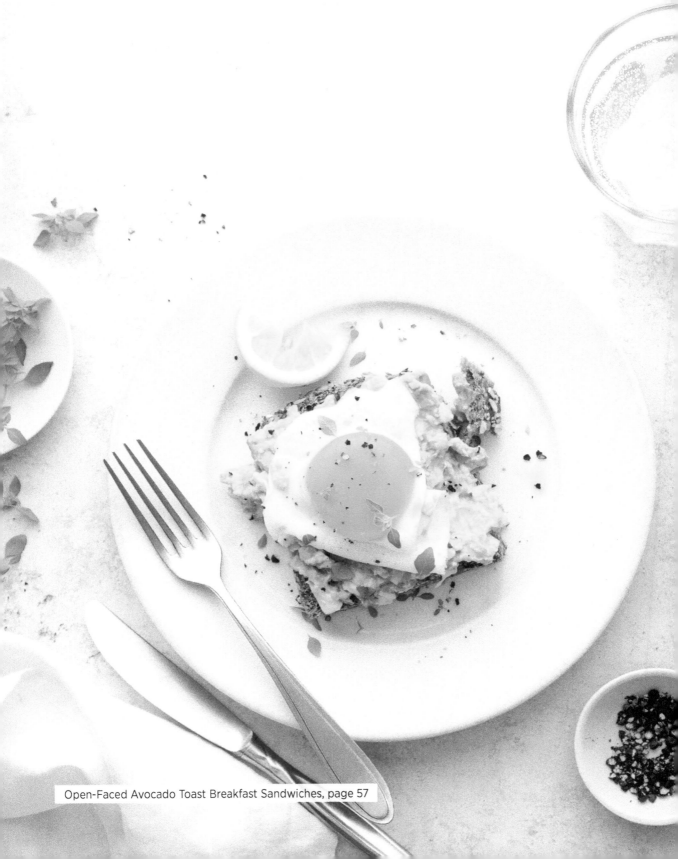

Open-Faced Avocado Toast Breakfast Sandwiches, page 57

Breakfast & Smoothies

COCOA-ALMOND SMOOTHIE

Serves 4 · **Prep time:** 10 minutes

Whether you use a blender, a food processor, or an immersion blender, smoothies pack a nutritious punch for a fast and easy breakfast on the go during busy weekday mornings. This version has almond butter, for plenty of protein, and high-antioxidant dark cocoa powder. Refrigerate or freeze extra servings and give them a quick blend the next morning.

4 cups unsweetened plain almond milk or nondairy milk of choice

1 cup crushed ice

3 tablespoons almond butter

2 tablespoons unsweetened cocoa powder

2 tablespoons honey or 4 stevia packets (to make vegan)

2 tablespoons chia seeds or flaxseed

½ teaspoon vanilla extract

In a blender or food processor, combine the almond milk, ice, almond butter, cocoa powder, honey, chia seeds, and vanilla. Blend until smooth.

Substitution tip: Feel free to use any low-fat milk that you enjoy here, such as skim milk, plain unsweetened rice milk, or soymilk.

Per serving: *Calories: 178; Total Fat: 11g; Saturated Fat: 1g; Cholesterol: 0mg; Carbohydrates: 18g; Fiber: 5g; Protein: 5g*

Gluten-free, Nut-free, Vegetarian

PUMPKIN SPICE SMOOTHIE

Serves 4 · **Prep time:** 10 minutes

If you can't wait for fall to start enjoying pumpkin spice–flavored everything, then this is the smoothie for you! Use canned pumpkin puree—NOT pumpkin pie mix, which has sugar and other spices already added. Sweeten with pure maple syrup, not imitation maple-flavored syrup.

4 cups skim milk
(to make nut-free)
or unsweetened plain
almond milk

1¼ cups canned
pumpkin puree

1 cup crushed ice

½ cup nonfat
Greek yogurt

¼ cup pure
maple syrup

1 teaspoon pumpkin
pie spice

In a blender or food processor, combine the milk, pumpkin puree, ice, yogurt, maple syrup, and pumpkin pie spice. Blend until smooth.

Substitution tip: Can't find pumpkin pie spice? Make your own with ½ teaspoon of cinnamon, ¼ teaspoon of nutmeg, and ¼ teaspoon of ground ginger.

Per serving: *Calories: 180; Total Fat: 1g; Saturated Fat: <1g; Cholesterol: 6mg; Carbohydrates: 33g; Fiber: 2g; Protein: 12g*

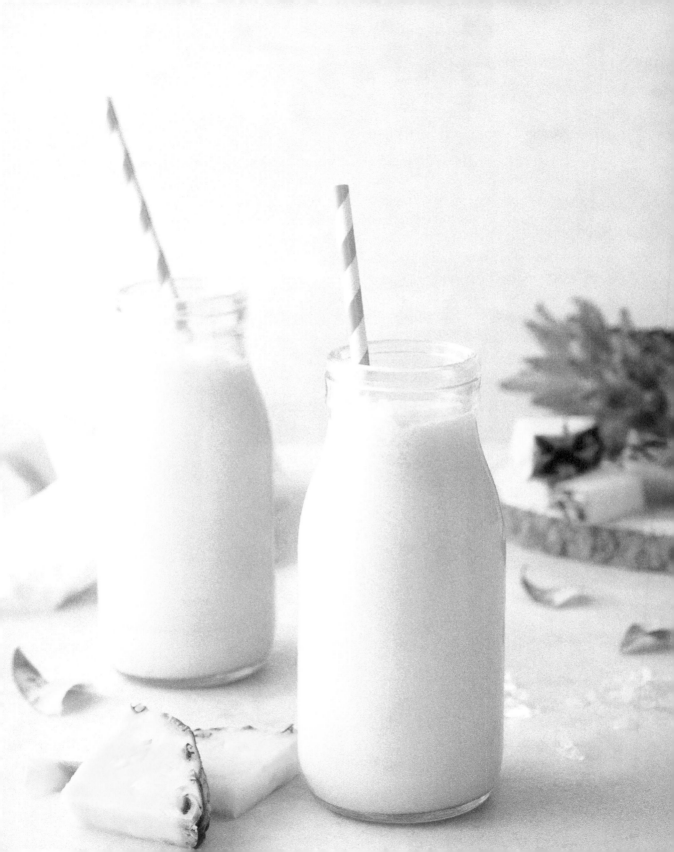

Dairy-free, Gluten-free, Vegan

PIÑA COLADA SMOOTHIE

Serves 4 · **Prep time:** 10 minutes

Transport yourself to a tropical paradise and make your morning just a bit better. This piña colada–flavored smoothie is sweet and slightly tropical, and it contains healthy fats and fresh pineapple, which is filled with digestive enzymes to help you fully digest your food.

2 cups chopped fresh pineapple

1 (13.5-ounce) can lite coconut milk

1 cup crushed ice

2 tablespoons flaxseed or chia seeds

½ teaspoon rum-flavored extract (optional)

In a blender or food processor, combine the pineapple, coconut milk, ice, flaxseed, and rum extract (if using). Blend until smooth.

Time-saving tip: Many grocery stores now have precut, fresh pineapple available, or you can purchase frozen (sugar-free) pineapple or even canned pineapple chunks in juice. Drain the canned chunks before using. If using frozen, omit the crushed ice.

Per serving: *Calories: 128; Total Fat: 7g; Saturated Fat: 5g; Cholesterol: 8mg; Carbohydrates: 15g; Fiber: 2g; Protein: 2g*

Gluten-free, Vegetarian

GREEK YOGURT AND BERRY PARFAIT

Serves 4 · **Prep time:** 10 minutes

You can put this breakfast together the night before and refrigerate it to allow the flavors to blend, or make it fresh in the morning. The Greek yogurt has lots of protein, while berries are high in antioxidants and add a tasty sweetness that balances the yogurt's tang.

2 cups nonfat or low-fat plain Greek yogurt

1 cup blueberries

1 cup sliced strawberries

1 cup raspberries

¼ cup pepitas

Divide the yogurt into 4 bowls. Sprinkle with the berries and top with the pepitas.

Substitution tip: Use any fresh, seasonally available berries. You can substitute blackberries, marionberries, or even cooked cranberries for any of the berries in this recipe.

Per serving: *Calories: 164; Total Fat: 5g; Saturated Fat: 1g; Cholesterol: 6mg; Carbohydrates: 17g; Fiber: 4g; Protein: 16g*

OVERNIGHT MAPLE-GINGER CHIA PUDDING

Serves 4 · **Prep time:** 10 minutes

Maple and ginger are a delicious flavor combination; the maple adds sweetness while the ginger adds a lovely bit of spice and heat. The chia seeds will thicken up when they sit in the liquid overnight, giving this pudding a nice, thick texture.

2 cups unsweetened plain almond milk or nondairy milk of choice

½ cup chia seeds

3 tablespoons pure maple syrup

2 teaspoons peeled and grated fresh ginger

½ teaspoon vanilla extract

1. In a mixing bowl, whisk together the almond milk, chia seeds, maple syrup, ginger, and vanilla.

2. Spoon into four bowls or small mason jars and refrigerate overnight.

Substitution tip: Turmeric has anti-inflammatory properties and adds a nice spice to this pudding as well. If you can find fresh turmeric (in the produce aisle near the ginger), feel free to replace the ginger with grated fresh turmeric.

Per serving: *Calories: 181; Total Fat: 8g; Saturated Fat: <1g; Cholesterol: 0mg; Carbohydrates: 22g; Fiber: 10g; Protein: 5g*

CRANBERRY-CINNAMON OVERNIGHT OATS

Serves 4 · **Prep time:** 10 minutes

Any time you can make something the night before and simply dig in the next morning on your way out the door, you've got a winner of a breakfast, particularly if it also uses nutritious ingredients like oats, chia, and fruit. This recipe hits all those high points, and it's quick, easy, and delicious.

2 cups skim milk

1½ cups old-
  fashioned oats

1 cup nonfat plain
  Greek yogurt

3 tablespoons pure
  maple syrup
  or honey

2 tablespoons
  chia seeds

½ teaspoon ground
  cinnamon

½ cup dried
  cranberries

1. In a mixing bowl, whisk together the milk, oats, yogurt, syrup, chia seeds, and cinnamon.

2. Fold in the cranberries.

3. Spoon into 4 bowls and refrigerate overnight. Serve cold.

Substitution tip: Oats might be processed on equipment that processes gluten grains, so they aren't necessarily gluten-free. Make sure that you use certified gluten-free oats if you have a gluten intolerance.

Per serving: *Calories: 321; Total Fat: 5g; Saturated Fat: 1g; Cholesterol: 6mg; Carbohydrates: 58g; Fiber: 7g; Protein: 15g*

Dairy-free, Gluten-free, Vegetarian

BANANA PANCAKES WITH WARM ALMOND BUTTER

Serves 4 · **Prep time:** 10 minutes · **Cook time:** 10 minutes

Ready to make the world's easiest pancakes? These are grain-free pancakes with tons of flavor, and you can top them with almond butter for even more flavor and protein. Be sure to spray your nonstick cooking pan liberally with nonstick cooking spray to help give the pancakes a crisp exterior.

Nonstick cooking spray

2 ripe bananas, peeled

4 large eggs, beaten

1 teaspoon
  ground nutmeg

¼ teaspoon
  baking powder

8 tablespoons
  almond butter

1. Preheat a large nonstick skillet or sauté pan on medium-high and spray it with cooking spray.

2. In a medium bowl, mash the bananas well.

3. Whisk in the eggs, nutmeg, and baking powder.

4. Drop in 2-tablespoon portions into the hot pan. Cook for 1 to 2 minutes per side, until just browned.

5. Serve, spread with the almond butter.

Troubleshooting tip: The biggest issue people tend to experience with these pancakes is that they are hard to flip if you make them too big, so stick to smaller pancakes, making about 16 small pancakes. To determine when they're browned, use your spatula to lift a corner of the pancake and take a peek.

Per serving (4 pancakes): *Calories 325; Total Fat: 23g; Saturated Fat: 3g; Cholesterol: 187mg; Carbohydrates: 20g; Fiber: 5g; Protein: 14g*

OATMEAL-RAISIN BREAKFAST COOKIES

Makes 8 cookies · **Prep time:** 10 minutes · **Cook time:** 15 minutes

What makes a breakfast cookie different from a regular cookie? For starters, it's low in sugar and more muffin-like in texture. It's a fast and easy breakfast, and you can even make a double or triple batch and keep them in the freezer for when you need breakfast or a snack in a hurry.

2 cups old-
  fashioned oats

2 very ripe
  bananas, mashed

½ cup almond butter

¼ cup raisins

1 large egg, beaten

½ teaspoon
  ground nutmeg

1. Preheat the oven to 350°F. Line a baking sheet with parchment paper.

2. In a medium bowl, mix the oats, bananas, almond butter, raisins, egg, and nutmeg until well combined.

3. Spoon onto the prepared baking sheet in 2-tablespoon mounds and flatten with a spatula.

4. Bake for about 10 minutes, until browned and set.

5. Cool slightly before serving. Store in an air-tight container for up to 4 days or freeze for up to 6 months.

Troubleshooting tip: Don't skip flattening these cookies, because they won't flatten by themselves. Flatten into your desired cookie shape before baking or you'll wind up with mounds instead of cookies.

Per serving (2 cookies): *Calories: 442; Total Fat: 22g; Saturated Fat: 2g; Cholesterol: 47mg; Carbohydrates: 54g; Fiber: 9g; Protein: 14g*

QUINOA, OAT, AND APRICOT BREAKFAST BARS

Serves 4 · **Prep time:** 10 minutes · **Cook time:** 20 minutes

With a texture similar to a soft granola bar, these spiced baked breakfast bars are delicious warm or cool. If you have another favorite dried fruit that you prefer, such as dried apples or cranberries, feel free to use it in place of the dried apricots.

1 cup cooked quinoa

½ cup old-fashioned oats

½ cup skim milk or unsweetened plain nondairy milk of choice

1 large egg, beaten

2 tablespoons almond butter, melted

1 tablespoon pure maple syrup

½ teaspoon ground cinnamon

Pinch sea salt

½ cup chopped dried apricots

1. Preheat the oven to 350°F. Line a bread pan with parchment paper.

2. In a medium bowl, mix the quinoa, oats, milk, egg, almond butter, syrup, cinnamon, and salt until well combined.

3. Fold in the apricots. Spread in the prepared pan.

4. Bake for about 20 minutes, until browned and set.

5. Slice into 4 pieces to serve. Store the bars in an airtight container in the refrigerator for up to 4 days or in the freezer for up to 6 months.

Substitution tip: If you have a nut allergy, you can replace the almond butter with an equal amount of any seed butter.

Per serving: *Calories: 225; Total Fat: 8g; Saturated Fat: 1g; Cholesterol: 47mg; Carbohydrates: 34g; Fiber: 4g; Protein: 8g*

Dairy-free, Nut-free, Vegetarian

WHOLE-GRAIN BANANA MUFFINS

Makes 12 muffins · **Prep** time: 10 minutes · **Cook** time: 25 minutes

The oats and whole-wheat flour in these muffins not only add lots of fiber, but they also make them filling and satisfying. This recipe yields 12 muffins, so feel free to freeze leftovers for quick breakfasts or snacks.

3 very ripe
   bananas, mashed

⅓ cup avocado oil or
   light olive oil

¼ cup pure
   maple syrup

¼ cup unsweetened
   plain almond milk
   or nondairy milk
   of choice

2 large eggs, beaten

1 teaspoon vanilla
   extract

1¾ cups whole-
   wheat flour

¼ cup old-
   fashioned oats

1 teaspoon
   baking soda

½ teaspoon ground
   cinnamon

1. Preheat the oven to 325°F. Line a 12-cup muffin tin with cupcake liners.

2. In a medium bowl, whisk together the bananas, oil, maple syrup, milk, eggs, and vanilla.

3. In another bowl, whisk together the flour, oats, baking soda, and cinnamon.

4. Add the wet ingredients to the dry and fold until just combined; there will still be some streaks of flour remaining in the batter.

5. Pour into the prepared muffin tins.

6. Bake for 20 to 25 minutes, until a toothpick inserted in the center of a muffin comes out clean.

7. Cool on wire racks before removing from the muffin tins. Store in an airtight container for up to 5 days or in the freezer for up to 6 months.

Substitution tip: Make pumpkin muffins by replacing the bananas with 1 cup of pumpkin puree and increasing the cinnamon to 1 teaspoon. Add ½ teaspoon of ginger and ¼ teaspoon of nutmeg for extra spice.

Per serving (1 muffin): *Calories: 177; Total Fat: 8g; Saturated Fat: 1g; Cholesterol: 31mg; Carbohydrates: 25g; Fiber: 3g; Protein: 4g*

Dairy-free, Nut-free, Vegetarian

OPEN-FACED AVOCADO TOAST BREAKFAST SANDWICHES

Serves 4 · **Prep time:** 10 minutes · **Cook time:** 5 minutes

Make eggs any way to go on these breakfast sandwiches; scrambled is the easiest, but you can also make them sunny-side up or over easy if you prefer. This breakfast is high in protein, and the fat in the avocado will keep you satiated throughout the morning, so you don't need a mid-morning snack.

1 tablespoon extra-virgin olive oil

4 large eggs, beaten

1 avocado, pitted, peeled, and mashed

Juice of ½ lemon

¼ teaspoon sea salt

4 slices whole-grain bread, toasted

1. In a nonstick skillet or sauté pan, heat the olive oil on medium until it shimmers.

2. Add the eggs and cook for about 5 minutes, scrambling, until set.

3. In a small bowl, combine the avocado, lemon juice, and salt. Mix well.

4. Spread the avocado mixture on the toast and top with the scrambled eggs.

Variation tip: If tomatoes are in season, add a big slice of fresh heirloom tomato on the avocado toast before you spoon the eggs on top.

Per serving: *Calories: 274; Total Fat: 16g; Saturated Fat: 3g; Cholesterol: 187mg; Carbohydrates: 22g; Fiber: 5g; Protein: 13g*

Dairy-free, Gluten-free, Nut-free, Vegan

SOUTHWEST TOFU SCRAMBLE

Serves 4 · **Prep time:** 10 minutes · **Cook time:** 10 minutes

This vegan breakfast scramble makes a nice change of pace from eggs. Use extra-firm tofu for the scramble, because it will hold its shape best. It's high in protein and moderate in fat, so it's a nutritious, stick-to-your ribs breakfast.

2 tablespoons extra-virgin olive oil

½ red onion, chopped

1 jalapeño pepper, seeds and ribs removed, chopped

1 pint cherry tomatoes, halved

8 ounces extra-firm tofu, cut into ½-inch pieces

½ teaspoon sea salt

½ teaspoon chili powder

½ teaspoon ground cumin

½ avocado, pitted, peeled, and chopped

¼ cup chopped fresh cilantro

1. In a nonstick skillet or sauté pan, heat the olive oil on medium-high until it shimmers. Add the onion and jalapeño and cook for about 5 minutes, stirring occasionally, until the vegetables soften.

2. Add the tomatoes, tofu, salt, chili powder, and cumin. Cook for about 5 minutes, stirring occasionally, until the tofu is heated through.

3. Remove from the heat and stir in the avocado and cilantro.

Time-saving tip: Replace the tomatoes and jalapeño with ½ cup of jarred salsa. Add in step 2 along with the tofu.

Per serving: *Calories: 170; Total Fat: 13g; Saturated Fat: 2g; Cholesterol: 0mg; Carbohydrates: 8g; Fiber: 3g; Protein: 7g*

Dairy-free, Nut-free, Vegan

VEGETARIAN BREAKFAST BURRITO

Serves 4 · **Prep time:** 15 minutes · **Cook time:** 25 minutes

You can make additional breakfast burritos by doubling this recipe. Then wrap in foil and freeze each in its own resealable bag. Reheat in the oven on 450°F, wrapped in foil, for about 15 minutes.

1 tablespoon extra-virgin olive oil

½ red onion, chopped

2 garlic cloves, minced

6 large eggs, beaten

1 cup canned black beans, drained and rinsed

½ teaspoon salt

4 (10-inch) whole-wheat tortillas

½ cup jarred salsa

1. Preheat the oven to 350°F.

2. In a large, nonstick skillet or sauté pan, heat the olive oil on medium-high until it shimmers. Add the onion and cook for about 5 minutes, stirring occasionally, until soft.

3. Add the garlic and cook, stirring constantly, for 30 seconds, until fragrant.

4. Add the eggs and cook for about 3 minutes, stirring, until set.

5. Add the black beans and salt and cook, stirring, for another 2 minutes, until heated through.

6. Spoon the egg mixture onto the tortillas and top with the salsa. Wrap and place, seam-side down, on a rimmed baking sheet. Bake for 20 minutes, then serve.

Serving tip: You can also sprinkle up to 2 tablespoons of shredded cheese per burrito on the filling before wrapping and baking.

Per serving: *Calories: 423; Total Fat: 17g; Saturated Fat: 5g; Cholesterol: 280mg; Carbohydrates: 50g; Fiber: 9g; Protein: 20g*

Gluten-free, Nut-free, Vegetarian

MUSHROOM AND SPINACH FRITTATA

Serves 4 · **Prep time:** 10 minutes · **Cook time:** 15 minutes

Frittatas are super easy to make and easy to customize with your own favorite veggies and herbs. This simple version pairs nutritious and meaty shiitake mushrooms with fresh baby spinach, cherry tomatoes, and fresh basil for a flavorful egg-based dish.

2 tablespoons extra-virgin olive oil

8 ounces sliced shiitake mushrooms

½ teaspoon sea salt

⅛ teaspoon freshly ground black pepper

2 cups fresh baby spinach

2 garlic cloves, minced

8 large eggs, beaten

2 tablespoons shredded Parmesan cheese (optional)

10 cherry tomatoes, halved

10 basil leaves, cut into strips

1. Preheat the broiler on high.

2. In a 10-inch, ovenproof skillet or sauté pan, heat the olive oil on medium-high until it shimmers.

3. Add the mushrooms, salt, and pepper. Cook for 5 to 7 minutes, stirring occasionally, until the mushrooms are browned.

4. Add the spinach and cook for about 2 minutes more, stirring, until just wilted.

5. Add the garlic and cook, stirring constantly, for 30 seconds, until fragrant.

6. Carefully pour the eggs over the vegetables. Cook without stirring, until the eggs set around the edge. Using a spatula, carefully pull the eggs away from the edge and tilt the pan to allow uncooked eggs to run into the spaces. Cook until set around the edges again.

7. Sprinkle with the Parmesan (if using) and arrange the cherry tomato halves and basil strips on the top.

8. Place the skillet under the broiler. Broil for about 4 minutes, until the top is browned. Slice into wedges to serve.

Technique tip: To cut the basil into strips, stack the leaves, roll them, and then slice into thin strips.

Per serving: *Calories: 248; Total Fat: 18g; Saturated Fat: 4g; Cholesterol: 373mg; Carbohydrates: 8g; Fiber: 2g; Protein: 15g*

Dairy-free, Gluten-free, Nut-free, Vegetarian

SHAKSHUKA

Serves 4 · **Prep time:** 10 minutes · **Cook time:** 25 minutes

Shakshuka is a Mediterranean-inspired tomato and egg dish that's bursting with flavor. It's also quick and easy to make, and it's a hearty, meat-free breakfast that's sure to please your whole family.

2 tablespoons
extra-virgin olive oil

1 red bell pepper,
chopped

½ yellow onion,
chopped

3 garlic cloves, minced

1 (28-ounce) can
crushed tomatoes

1 teaspoon paprika

½ teaspoon
ground cumin

½ teaspoon sea salt

⅛ teaspoon freshly
ground black pepper

4 large eggs

1. Preheat the oven to 375°F.

2. In a 12-inch ovenproof skillet or sauté pan, heat the olive oil on medium-high until it shimmers. Add the bell pepper and onion and cook for about 5 minutes, stirring occasionally, until the veggies are soft.

3. Add the garlic and cook, stirring constantly, for 30 seconds, until fragrant.

4. Add the tomatoes and their juices, paprika, cumin, salt, and black pepper. Bring to a simmer. Cook for about 10 minutes, stirring occasionally, until the sauce has thickened.

5. Carefully crack the eggs over the tomatoes. Spoon a little sauce around the edges, leaving the yolks exposed.

6. Transfer to the oven. Cook until the eggs set, about 10 minutes more.

Serving tip: Before serving, sprinkle with 2 tablespoons of chopped fresh oregano and 2 tablespoons of crumbled feta cheese.

Per serving: *Calories: 224; Total Fat: 13g; Saturated Fat: 3g; Cholesterol: 187mg; Carbohydrates: 20g; Fiber: 5g; Protein: 11g*

Dairy-free, Gluten-free, Nut-free

SALMON SCRAMBLE

Serves 4 · **Prep time:** 5 minutes · **Cook time:** 15 minutes

Salmon is packed with nutritious, anti-inflammatory omega-3 fatty acids, and it adds delicious flavor to this simple scramble. Use water-packed, wild-caught Pacific salmon from either a pouch or a can because it's much more nutritious than Atlantic salmon.

1 tablespoon extra-virgin olive oil

½ red onion, chopped

1 (2.5-ounce) pouch wild-caught salmon, rinsed and drained

2 tablespoons capers, drained and rinsed

6 large eggs, beaten

⅛ teaspoon freshly ground black pepper

2 tablespoons chopped fresh dill

1. In a large, nonstick skillet or sauté pan, heat the olive oil on medium-high until it shimmers.

2. Add the onion and cook for about 5 minutes, stirring occasionally, until soft.

3. Add the salmon and capers and cook, stirring, for 2 minutes more.

4. Add the eggs and pepper. Cook for 3 to 5 minutes more, scrambling, until the eggs are set.

5. Remove from the heat and stir in the dill.

Substitution tip: If you can't find chopped, fresh dill or if it isn't in season, you can use ½ teaspoon of dried dill. Add it with the salmon and capers in step 3.

Per serving: *Calories: 173; Total Fat: 12g; Saturated Fat: 3g; Cholesterol: 289mg; Carbohydrates: 2g; Fiber: <1g; Protein: 14g*

Dairy-free, Gluten-free, Nut-free

KALE, RED PEPPER, AND TURKEY BACON EGG CUPS

Makes 12 cups · **Prep time:** 15 minutes · **Cook time:** 35 minutes

These convenient "muffins" are superstars in the freezer. Make a double or triple batch, remove them from the muffin tins, and freeze them in single-serving sizes in zip-top bags. Reheat in a 350°F oven for about 20 minutes, or until heated through.

Nonstick cooking spray

3 tablespoons
 extra-virgin olive oil

6 slices turkey bacon

3 cups stemmed and
 chopped fresh kale

1 red bell pepper,
 chopped

2 garlic cloves, minced

12 large eggs, beaten

1½ tablespoons Dijon
 mustard

½ teaspoon sea salt

⅛ teaspoon freshly
 ground black pepper

Pinch red pepper
 flakes (optional)

1. Preheat the oven to 350°F. Spray 12 cups of a nonstick muffin tin with cooking spray.

2. In a nonstick skillet or sauté pan, heat the olive oil on medium-high until it shimmers. Add the bacon and cook for about 6 minutes, until browned. Drain and crumble.

3. In the same pan, cook the kale and bell pepper in the remaining oil for about 5 minutes, stirring occasionally, until the vegetables are soft. Add the garlic and cook, stirring constantly, for 30 seconds. Let cool.

4. In a medium bowl, whisk together the eggs, mustard, salt, black pepper, and red pepper flakes (if using) until well combined.

5. Divide the vegetables and crumbled bacon among the muffin cups. Carefully pour the eggs over the top.

6. Bake for about 20 minutes, until the eggs are just set. Store in an airtight container in the refrigerator for up to 3 days or in the freezer for up to 6 months.

Substitution tip: These cups are easily customizable to whatever vegetables you have on hand, just make sure to cook them until tender before adding. Zucchini, asparagus, mushrooms, and other greens like spinach all work nicely in these.

Per serving (2 muffins): *Calories: 280; Total Fat: 21g; Saturated Fat: 5g; Cholesterol: 394mg; Carbohydrates: 4g; Fiber: 1g; Protein: 17g*

TURKEY BREAKFAST SAUSAGE PATTIES

Serves 4 · **Prep time:** 5 minutes · **Cook time:** 10 minutes·

Enjoy these lower-fat but still highly flavorful sausage patties alongside some scrambled eggs for a complete breakfast, or eat them on whole-grain toast for a tasty breakfast sandwich. They're a great lower-fat, lower-calorie alternative to traditional pork breakfast sausage.

8 ounces ground turkey breast

1 teaspoon ground sage

½ teaspoon garlic powder

½ teaspoon sea salt

¼ teaspoon freshly ground black pepper

⅛ teaspoon red pepper flakes

2 tablespoons extra-virgin olive oil or nonstick cooking spray

1. In a large bowl, combine the turkey breast, sage, garlic powder, salt, black pepper, and red pepper flakes. Mix well.

2. Form into 8 patties.

3. In a nonstick skillet or sauté pan, heat the olive oil on medium-high until it shimmers. Cook the sausage for about 4 minutes per side, until browned.

Time-saving tip: You can also cook this meat as sausage crumbles; simply cook, crumbling with a spoon as you do, until browned, about 5 minutes. Then you can freeze in 2-ounce servings and use in scrambled eggs.

Per serving (2 patties): *Calories: 120; Total Fat: 7g; Saturated Fat: 1g; Cholesterol: 35mg; Carbohydrates: 0g; Fiber: 0g; Protein: 14g*

Gluten-free, Nut-free

MEXICAN-INSPIRED BREAKFAST CHILAQUILES

Serves 4 · **Prep time:** 10 minutes · **Cook time:** 15 minutes

This spicy breakfast is based on the Mexican-inspired comfort food chilaquiles, which are fried tortilla strips topped with cheese and salsa. This version is lighter, using crushed blue corn tortilla chips scrambled with eggs and topped with a light sprinkling of cotija cheese, which you can find in the dairy department of most grocery stores.

2 tablespoons extra-virgin olive oil

½ yellow onion, chopped

1 (2-ounce) can chopped chiles, drained

2 cups crushed baked blue corn chips or regular corn chips

8 large eggs, beaten

½ teaspoon sea salt

½ teaspoon chili powder

½ cup jarred salsa

¼ cup crumbled cotija cheese (optional)

¼ cup chopped fresh cilantro

1. In a large, nonstick skillet or sauté pan, heat the olive oil on medium-high until it shimmers. Add the onion and cook for 5 minutes, stirring occasionally, until soft.

2. Add the chiles and cook, stirring, for 2 minutes more, until heated through.

3. Add the tortilla chips and cook for 2 more minutes, stirring.

4. In a bowl, whisk together the eggs, salt, and chili powder. Add to the pan and cook for about 4 minutes, scrambling, until the eggs are set.

5. Add the salsa and cook, stirring, for 2 minutes more, until heated through.

6. Remove from the heat and sprinkle with the cheese (if using) and cilantro just before serving.

Per serving: Calories: 447; Total Fat: 27g; Saturated Fat: 5g; Cholesterol: 373mg; Carbohydrates: 36g; Fiber: 4g; Protein: 16g

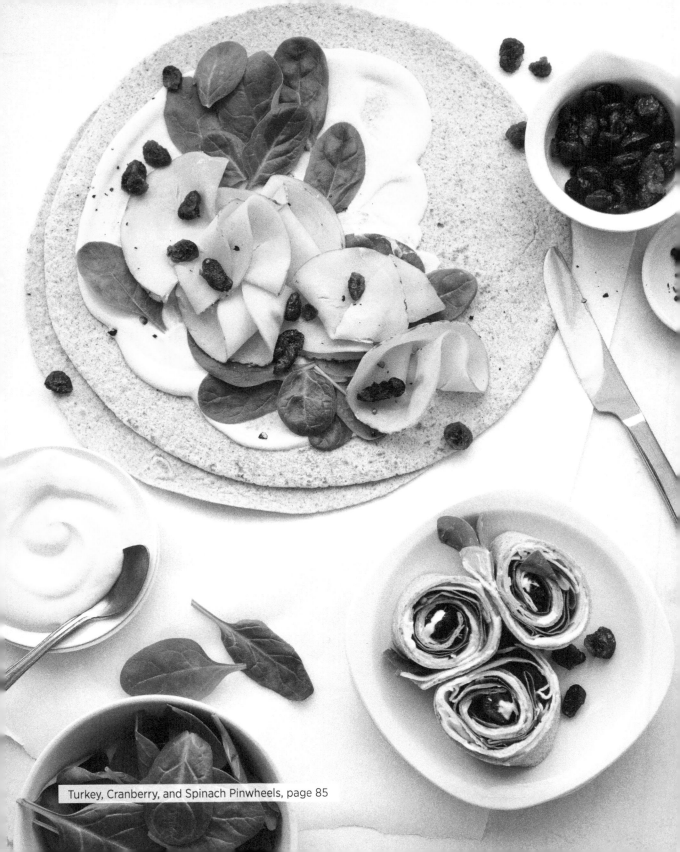

Turkey, Cranberry, and Spinach Pinwheels, page 85

Salads, Soups & Sandwiches

Dairy-free, Gluten-free, Vegan

STRAWBERRY AND SPINACH SALAD

Serves 4 · **Prep time:** 10 minutes

This salad is bright, colorful, and refreshing. Use an aged balsamic vinegar for best flavor, or you can substitute a flavored vinegar, such as fig or raspberry vinegar. The salad is high in fiber and thoroughly delicious.

6 cups fresh
   baby spinach

1 pint
   strawberries, sliced

¼ cup walnut pieces

¼ red onion,
   thinly sliced

¼ cup balsamic vinegar

¼ cup extra-virgin
   olive oil

1 teaspoon Dijon
   mustard

¼ teaspoon sea salt

⅛ teaspoon freshly
   ground black pepper

1. In a large bowl, combine the spinach, strawberries, walnuts, and red onion.

2. In a small bowl, whisk together the vinegar, olive oil, mustard, salt, and pepper. Toss with the salad.

Variation tip: Add a salty tang by garnishing the salad with 2 tablespoons of crumbled feta cheese before serving.

Per serving: *Calories: 220; Total Fat: 19g; Saturated Fat: 2g; Cholesterol: 0mg; Carbohydrates: 12g; Fiber: 3g; Protein: 3g*

Dairy-free, Gluten-free, Nut-free, Vegetarian

SWEET AND SPICY SLAW

Serves 4 · **Prep time:** 10 minutes

This crunchy, sweet-and-spicy slaw makes a refreshing side dish that's delicious with chicken or pork. You can even shred some cooked chicken breast and toss it with the slaw for a quick and easy meal. Store the slaw for up to 3 days in the refrigerator.

1 (16-ounce) bag
   tri-color coleslaw mix

6 scallions, both white
   and green parts,
   thinly sliced

¼ cup apple cider
   vinegar

¼ cup extra-virgin olive
   oil or avocado oil

1 tablespoon peeled
   and grated
   fresh ginger

1 tablespoon honey or
   1 stevia packet

2 garlic cloves, minced

½ teaspoon sriracha

½ teaspoon Chinese
   hot mustard

¼ teaspoon sea salt

1. In a large bowl, combine the coleslaw mix and scallions.

2. In a small bowl, whisk together the vinegar, olive oil, ginger, honey, garlic, sriracha, mustard, and salt.

3. Toss with the salad to mix.

Serving tip: For some added texture and flavor, sprinkle with 2 tablespoons of sesame seeds or chopped peanuts.

Per serving: *Calories: 176; Total Fat: 14g; Saturated Fat: 2g; Cholesterol: 0mg; Carbohydrates: 14g; Fiber: 3g; Protein: 2g*

SOUTHWEST-INSPIRED CORN AND AVOCADO SALAD

Serves 4 · **Prep time:** 10 minutes · **Cook time:** 10 minutes

If you have one, using an outdoor grill to cook the corn on the cob will impart a smoky flavor to this delicious summer salad. The result is a colorful, complex, and flavorful salad that will keep well in the refrigerator for up to 5 days.

4 corn cobs, husks and silks removed

1 pint cherry tomatoes, halved

1 avocado, pitted, peeled, and chopped

½ red onion, finely chopped

¼ cup chopped fresh cilantro

1 hatch chile pepper, seeds and ribs removed, finely chopped

Juice of 2 limes

2 tablespoons avocado oil

½ teaspoon sea salt

½ teaspoon chipotle chili powder

1. Heat a grill or grill pan on medium-high. Grill the corn for about 5 minutes, turning frequently, until browned. Let cool.

2. When the corn is cool, cut the kernels from the cob and place them in a large bowl.

3. Add the cherry tomatoes, avocado, red onion, cilantro, and chile pepper.

4. In a small bowl, whisk together the lime juice, avocado oil, salt, and chili powder. Toss with the salad.

Variation tip: Make this a full meal by adding 8 ounces of cooked baby shrimp to the salad.

Per serving: *Calories: 242; Total Fat: 14g; Saturated Fat: 2g; Cholesterol: 0mg; Carbohydrates: 31g; Fiber: 6g; Protein: 5g*

Dairy-free, Gluten-free, Nut-free, Vegan

THREE-BEAN SALAD

Serves 4 · **Prep time:** 10 minutes · **Cook time:** 5 minutes

Blanching the green beans beforehand softens them and helps maintain a bright green color that makes this salad visually appetizing. You can store this salad for up to 4 days in the refrigerator before serving; the longer you refrigerate it, the better the flavors mix.

2 cups fresh green beans, halved

1 (15-ounce) can kidney beans, drained and rinsed

1 (15-ounce) can chickpeas, drained and rinsed

½ red onion, thinly sliced

¼ cup chopped fresh Italian parsley

¼ cup red wine vinegar

¼ cup extra-virgin olive oil

1 teaspoon Dijon mustard

2 garlic cloves, minced

¼ teaspoon sea salt

1. Bring a large pot of water to a boil and prepare a large bowl with ice water. Add the green beans to the boiling water and cook for 2 minutes. Plunge the beans into ice water to stop the cooking. Drain.

2. In another large bowl, combine the green beans, kidney beans, chickpeas, red onion, and parsley. Mix.

3. In a small bowl, whisk together the vinegar, olive oil, mustard, garlic, and salt.

4. Toss the beans with the dressing, mixing well. Refrigerate for about 30 minutes before serving to allow the flavors to mix.

Technique tip: If you find the flavor of red onions too strong, soak the sliced onions in cold water for about 20 minutes and then pat them dry before adding them to the salad.

Per serving: *Calories: 337; Total Fat: 16g; Saturated Fat: 2g; Cholesterol: 0mg; Carbohydrates: 37g; Fiber: 10g; Protein: 12g*

Dairy-free, Gluten-free, Nut-free

ITALIAN-INSPIRED CHOPPED SALAD

Serves 4 · **Prep time:** 10 minutes

You can pick up a rotisserie chicken at the grocery store or precooked chicken breast to make this meal salad quick and easy. Alternatively, cook boneless, skinless chicken breasts, chop them, and store in freezer bags in 1-cup servings for use in recipes to save time.

2 cups cooked, cooled, and chopped boneless, skinless chicken breast

1 (15-ounce) can water-packed artichoke hearts, drained and chopped

1 red bell pepper, chopped

½ red onion, chopped

¼ cup red wine vinegar

¼ cup extra-virgin olive oil

1 teaspoon Dijon mustard

1 teaspoon dried oregano

3 garlic cloves, minced

¼ teaspoon sea salt

⅛ teaspoon freshly ground black pepper

1. In a large bowl, mix the chicken, artichoke hearts, bell pepper, and onion.

2. In a smaller bowl, whisk together the vinegar, olive oil, mustard, oregano, garlic, salt, and black pepper.

3. Toss the dressing with the salad and mix well.

Substitution tip: This also works well with water-packed canned tuna or salmon in place of the chicken, which adds healthy omega-3 fatty acids.

Per serving: *Calories: 265; Total Fat: 15g; Saturated Fat: 2g; Cholesterol: 45mg; Carbohydrates: 10g; Fiber: 4g; Protein: 20g*

Dairy-free, Gluten-free, Nut-free

CHICKEN COBB SALAD

Serves 4 · **Prep time:** 10 minutes · **Cook time:** 5 minutes

This pared-down version of a Cobb salad includes the classic flavors but omits the high-fat, salty blue cheese. To store, keep the dressing and salad separate so it doesn't get soggy. It will keep in the refrigerator for up to 3 days.

6 cups shredded Romaine lettuce

2 cups cooked, cooled, and chopped boneless, skinless chicken breast

1 pint cherry tomatoes, halved

2 slices turkey bacon, browned and crumbled

2 hard-boiled eggs, peeled and chopped

¼ cup low-fat mayonnaise or low-fat plain Greek yogurt

¼ cup skim milk, nondairy milk, or low-fat buttermilk

2 tablespoons Dijon mustard

1 tablespoon honey

¼ teaspoon sea salt

1. In a large bowl, combine the lettuce, chicken, tomatoes, bacon, and eggs.

2. In a smaller bowl, whisk together the mayonnaise, milk, mustard, honey, and salt. Toss with the salad.

Technique tip: To hard-boil eggs, place them in the bottom of a saucepan and cover with cold water that goes an inch over the top of the eggs. Place on a cool burner, turn the heat to high, and bring to a boil. As soon as the water boils, turn off the heat, cover the pot, and allow to sit off the heat for 14 minutes. Then plunge the eggs into ice water to cool them. This should help you peel the eggs more quickly, but if you're still having trouble, run them under cold water as you peel. Likewise, eggs that are slightly older (a week or two) are much easier to peel when hard-boiled than fresh eggs.

Per serving: *Calories: 239; Total Fat: 10g; Saturated Fat: 2g; Cholesterol: 141mg; Carbohydrates: 13g; Fiber: 3g; Protein: 24g*

Dairy-free, Gluten-free, Nut-free, Vegan

SPICY GAZPACHO

Serves 4 · **Prep time:** 10 minutes

This chilled vegetable soup makes a light, refreshing lunch or snack. Use the freshest tomatoes you can find for the best flavor, and puree to your desired consistency in a blender or food processor. Gazpacho will store in the refrigerator for up to 3 days, but it will taste better fresh.

4 large heirloom tomatoes, chopped

1 cucumber, chopped

1 red bell pepper, chopped

1 shallot, chopped

¼ cup extra-virgin olive oil

2 tablespoons red wine vinegar

10 fresh basil leaves, torn

2 garlic cloves, peeled and chopped

½ teaspoon sea salt

¼ teaspoon freshly ground black pepper

1. In a blender or food processor, combine the tomatoes, cucumber, bell pepper, shallot, olive oil, vinegar, basil, garlic, salt, and black pepper. Blend until smooth.

2. Chill for 2 hours before serving.

Serving tip: Add some crunch by topping each serving of soup with 2 tablespoons of roasted pepitas.

Per serving: *Calories: 182; Total Fat: 14g; Saturated Fat: 2g; Cholesterol: 0mg; Carbohydrates: 14g; Fiber: 4g; Protein: 3g*

Dairy-free, Gluten-free, Nut-free, Vegan

MINESTRONE

Serves 4 · **Prep time:** 15 minutes · **Cook time:** 30 minutes

This Italian-inspired veggie soup is warming and flavorful. It freezes extremely well; you can freeze it in single 1-cup servings for up to 6 months or store it in the refrigerator for up to 5 days.

2 tablespoons extra-virgin olive oil

1 yellow onion, chopped

1 zucchini, chopped

4 garlic cloves, minced

6 cups low-sodium vegetable broth

2 cups green beans, cut into 1-inch pieces

1 (14.5-ounce) can crushed tomatoes

1 tablespoon dried Italian herbs

½ teaspoon sea salt

⅛ teaspoon freshly ground black pepper

1. In a large pot, heat the olive oil on medium-high until it shimmers. Add the onion and zucchini and cook for about 5 minutes, stirring occasionally, until the veggies soften.

2. Add the garlic and cook, stirring constantly, for 30 seconds, until fragrant.

3. Add the broth, green beans, tomatoes and their juices, Italian herbs, salt, and pepper. Bring to a simmer, stirring occasionally. Reduce the heat and simmer for 20 minutes, stirring occasionally, until the flavors meld.

Substitution tip: For more flavor, add crushed or chopped fire-roasted tomatoes with basil in place of the crushed tomatoes.

Per serving: *Calories: 150; Total Fat: 7g; Saturated Fat: 1g; Cholesterol: 0mg; Carbohydrates: 20g; Fiber: 5g; Protein: 4g*

Dairy-free, Nut-free

CHICKEN NOODLE SOUP

Serves 4 · **Prep time:** 15 minutes · **Cook time:** 25 minutes

Is there any soup that's more of a comfort food than chicken noodle soup? This simple chicken soup recipe will remind you of Mom's, and with the benefit of adaptability you can make it gluten-free, use more garlic if you prefer, add a pinch of red pepper flakes for spice, or even add a squeeze of lemon juice at the end of cooking for some acidity.

2 tablespoons extra-virgin olive oil

8 ounces boneless, skinless chicken breast, cut into ½-inch pieces

1 yellow onion, chopped

1 red bell pepper, chopped

2 carrots, peeled and chopped

2 garlic cloves, minced

6 cups low-sodium chicken broth

3 ounces dried whole-wheat spaghetti noodles or gluten-free spaghetti noodles

½ teaspoon sea salt

¼ teaspoon freshly ground black pepper

1. In a large pot, heat the olive oil on medium-high until it shimmers. Add the chicken and cook for about 7 minutes, stirring occasionally, until it is opaque. Using a slotted spoon, remove the chicken from the fat in the pot, and set it aside.

2. Add the onion, bell pepper, and carrots to the pot. Cook for about 5 minutes, stirring occasionally, until the veggies soften. Add the garlic and cook for 30 seconds, stirring constantly, until fragrant.

3. Add the chicken broth and bring to a simmer. Return the chicken and any juices to the pot. Add the noodles, salt, and black pepper. Simmer for 12 minutes, stirring occasionally, until the noodles are tender.

Substitution tip: You can make this gluten-free by either using gluten-free noodles or replacing the noodles with one large zucchini, cut into noodles using a spiralizer or by peeling strips with a vegetable peeler and cutting each strip into noodle shapes.

Per serving: *Calories: 263; Total Fat: 10g; Saturated Fat: 1g; Cholesterol: 48mg; Carbohydrates: 26g; Fiber: 4g; Protein: 18g*

Dairy-free, Gluten-free, Nut-free, Vegan

ROASTED TOMATO AND RED PEPPER SOUP

Serves 4 · **Prep time:** 15 minutes · **Cook time:** 25 minutes

This simple soup uses canned fire-roasted tomatoes (Muir Glen makes a great organic version with lots of flavor) and jarred roasted peppers. See the technique tip for safe pureeing of the soup, because pureeing hot soup can be hazardous if you don't manage it correctly. This soup will keep in the refrigerator for up to 5 days or in the freezer for up to 6 months.

2 tablespoons extra-virgin olive oil

1 yellow onion, finely chopped

3 garlic cloves, minced

4 cups low-sodium vegetable broth

1 (28-ounce) can fire-roasted whole tomatoes

1 (15-ounce) jar roasted red peppers, drained and rinsed

½ teaspoon sea salt

¼ teaspoon red pepper flakes

⅛ teaspoon freshly ground black pepper

10 basil leaves, torn

1. In a large pot, heat the olive oil on medium-high until it shimmers. Add the onion and cook for about 5 minutes, stirring occasionally, until soft. Add the garlic and cook for 30 seconds, stirring constantly, until fragrant.

2. Add the broth, tomatoes and their juices, red peppers, salt, red pepper flakes, and black pepper. Bring to a simmer. Reduce the heat to medium and cook for 10 minutes, stirring occasionally, until the flavors meld.

3. Remove from the heat. Stir in the basil. Use an immersion blender or transfer to a blender or food processor and puree until smooth.

Technique tip: To safely puree hot soup in a blender or food processor, pour into the processing container and put the lid on. Fold a towel and place it over the top of the processor or blender to protect your hand. Place your hand on top of the towel. Puree for about 10 seconds, and then carefully lift the lid away from your face to allow steam to escape. Put the top back on, put the towel back in place, and puree again. Do this in 10- to 20-second increments until the soup reaches the desired consistency.

Per serving: *Calories: 181; Total Fat: 7g; Saturated Fat: 1g; Cholesterol: 0mg; Carbohydrates: 27g; Fiber: 6g; Protein: 6g*

CREAMY CLAM CHOWDER

Serves 4 · **Prep time:** 10 minutes · **Cook time:** 25 minutes

If you're a fan of New England clam chowder, then you'll like this lightened-up version. This has options to be gluten-free and dairy-free.

2 tablespoons extra-virgin olive oil

3 slices peppered turkey bacon, chopped

1 yellow onion, finely chopped

2 carrots, peeled and chopped

1 fennel bulb, cored and chopped, plus 2 tablespoons chopped fennel fronds, divided

3 tablespoons whole-wheat flour or gluten-free all-purpose flour

6 cups low-sodium vegetable broth

1 (6.5-ounce) can clams

½ teaspoon sea salt

¼ cup skim milk or unsweetened plain nondairy milk

1. In a large pot, heat the olive oil on medium-high until it shimmers. Add the bacon and cook for about 5 minutes, until browned. Using a slotted spoon, remove the bacon from the fat and set aside.

2. Add the onion, carrots, and fennel bulb to the fat and cook for about 5 minutes, stirring occasionally, until the vegetables soften.

3. Add the flour and cook for 1 minute, stirring constantly.

4. Add the broth, clams and their juices, and salt. Return the bacon to the pot. Bring to a simmer, stirring frequently, and reduce the heat to medium low. Simmer, stirring frequently, for 10 minutes, until the flavors meld.

5. Stir in the milk and fennel fronds and cook, stirring, for 1 minute more, until heated through.

Substitution tip: Turn this into a vegan corn chowder by omitting the bacon and replacing the clams with a 14-ounce can of corn, drained. Add the corn when you would add the clams.

Per serving: *Calories: 208; Total Fat:9 g; Saturated Fat: 2g; Cholesterol: 26mg; Carbohydrates: 21g; Fiber: 5g; Protein: 11g*

Dairy-free, Gluten-free, Nut-free

GROUND BEEF AND CABBAGE SOUP

Serves 4 · **Prep time:** 10 minutes · **Cook time:** 25 minutes

Using extra-lean ground beef keeps this soup lower in fat, but it's definitely not short on flavor. The trick to making sure the soup has plenty of flavor is caramelizing the onions slowly on low heat until they develop a deep brown color and a rich flavor.

1 pound extra-lean ground beef

2 tablespoons extra-virgin olive oil

2 yellow onions, thinly sliced

2 garlic cloves, minced

6 cups low-sodium chicken broth

1 green cabbage head, shredded

1 (14.5-ounce) can chopped tomatoes

1 teaspoon Dijon mustard

1 teaspoon ground caraway

½ teaspoon sea salt

1. In a large pot, cook the beef on medium-high for about 5 minutes, crumbling with a spoon, until it is browned. Remove from the pot and set aside.

2. In the same pot, heat the olive oil until it shimmers. Add the onions and reduce the heat to low. Cook for about 15 minutes, stirring occasionally, until the onions are golden brown.

3. Add the garlic and cook, stirring constantly, for 30 seconds, until fragrant.

4. Add the broth, cabbage, tomatoes and their juices, mustard, caraway, and salt. Using the side of a spoon, scrape any browned bits from the bottom of the pan.

5. Return the ground beef to the pot. Turn the temperature up to medium-high and bring to a simmer, stirring occasionally. Simmer for 10 minutes until the flavors meld.

Substitution tip: You can make this vegetarian by using 16 ounces of vegetarian crumbles in place of the ground beef. If you do that, you can skip step 1.

Per serving: *Calories: 340; Total Fat: 12g; Saturated Fat: 3g; Cholesterol: 78mg; Carbohydrates: 27g; Fiber: 8g; Protein: 30g*

Dairy-free, Vegan

SPICY HUMMUS AND VEGGIE PITA

Serves 4 · **Prep time:** 15 minutes

You can either use my hummus recipe or save time by purchasing prepared hummus. The combination of spicy, creamy hummus and crunchy veggies makes this a delicious sandwich. If you're taking it to work, keep the hummus in a separate container until you're ready to eat the sandwich.

1 recipe Hummus and Red Bell Pepper Sticks (page 149)

¼ cup pine nuts

¼ teaspoon chili oil (optional)

4 whole-wheat pita halves

1 cup stemmed and chopped fresh kale

1. In a bowl, mix the hummus with the pine nuts and chili oil (if using).

2. Spread the inside of each pita half with the hummus.

3. Add the bell pepper sticks and the kale.

Serving tip: Want more crunch? Add a tablespoon of pepitas to the sandwich.

Per serving: *Calories: 324; Total Fat: 17g; Saturated Fat: 2g; Cholesterol: 0mg; Carbohydrates: 39g; Fiber: 9g; Protein: 10g*

Nut-free

DILLED TUNA SALAD SANDWICHES

Serves 4 · **Prep time:** 15 minutes

This is a lighter take on a traditional tuna salad sandwich, but the presence of fresh dill takes it to the next level. If you're storing the sandwich, keep the tuna salad separate from the bread and put it together just before you eat it.

2 (5-ounce) cans water-packed tuna, drained

1 (8-ounce) can sliced water chestnuts, drained and chopped

4 scallions, both white and green parts, thinly sliced

¼ cup chopped fresh dill

¼ cup nonfat plain Greek yogurt

1 teaspoon Dijon mustard

½ teaspoon sea salt

⅛ teaspoon freshly ground black pepper

8 slices whole-wheat bread

1. In a large bowl, combine the tuna, water chestnuts, scallions, and dill.

2. In another bowl, whisk together the yogurt, mustard, salt, and pepper. Toss with the tuna salad.

3. Spread on the bread to make 4 sandwiches.

Substitution tip: You can make this gluten-free by wrapping the tuna salad in large pieces of butter lettuce in place of the bread to create a lettuce wrap.

Per serving: *Calories: 305; Total Fat: 4g; Saturated Fat: 1g; Cholesterol: 24mg; Carbohydrates: 43g; Fiber: 6g; Protein: 26g*

Dairy-free, Nut-free

SHRIMP CEVICHE WRAPS

Serves 4 · **Prep time:** 15 minutes

This simple ceviche starts with cooked baby shrimp, so you don't need to rely on the citrus juices to "cook" the shrimp. You can use any combination of freshly squeezed citrus juices (orange, lime, and lemon make an excellent combo) to make this delicious wrap.

8 ounces cooked baby shrimp

1 pint cherry tomatoes, chopped

½ avocado, pitted, peeled, and chopped

½ red onion, chopped

¼ cup chopped fresh cilantro

1 garlic clove, minced

½ cup freshly squeezed citrus juice

½ teaspoon sea salt

4 (7-inch) whole-wheat tortillas

1. In a large bowl, combine the shrimp, tomatoes, avocado, onion, cilantro, and garlic.

2. Add the citrus juice and salt and mix well. Refrigerate for at least 30 minutes to allow the flavors to blend.

3. Before serving, divide the ceviche among the tortillas and wrap.

Substitution tip: Corn tortillas or large pieces of butter lettuce make this a gluten-free wrap if you need to watch your gluten intake.

Per serving: *Calories: 259; Total Fat: 7g; Saturated Fat: 2g; Cholesterol: 120mg; Carbohydrates: 32g; Fiber: 5g; Protein: 18g*

TURKEY, CRANBERRY, AND SPINACH PINWHEELS

Serves 4 · **Prep time:** 15 minutes

Pinwheel sandwiches are great meals for on the go. You can prepare them the night before and then grab one for a quick lunch. They'll keep in the refrigerator for up to 5 days.

¼ cup nonfat plain Greek yogurt

1 tablespoon Dijon mustard

¼ teaspoon sea salt

4 (7-inch) whole-wheat tortillas

8 ounces deli-sliced turkey breast

1 cup fresh baby spinach

¼ cup dried cranberries

1. In a small bowl, whisk together the yogurt, mustard, and salt. Spread on the tortillas.

2. Top with the turkey slices and spinach. Sprinkle with the dried cranberries and wrap.

3. Cut each wrap into 1- to 1½-inch pieces.

Substitution tip: Kale also works well in place of spinach in these sandwiches. Trim the leaves away from the ribs and use only the leaves.

Per serving: *Calories: 237; Total Fat: 5g; Saturated Fat: 1g; Cholesterol: 25mg; Carbohydrates: 32g; Fiber: 4g; Protein: 18g*

Nut-free

GREEK-INSPIRED CHICKEN SALAD PITAS

Serves 4 · **Prep time:** 15 minutes

Greek flavors add interest to a standard chicken salad, making it an enticing and delicious lunch sandwich. If you need to make it gluten-free, you can spoon the chicken salad into lettuce cups instead of into the pitas.

1 pint cherry tomatoes, halved

8 ounces cooked bone-less, skinless chicken breast, chopped

¼ cup chopped black olives

¼ cup nonfat or low-fat plain Greek yogurt

Zest and juice of ½ lemon

1 tablespoon Dijon mustard

1 garlic clove, minced

1 teaspoon dried oregano

4 whole-wheat pita halves

1. In a large bowl, mix the tomatoes, chicken, and olives.

2. In another bowl, whisk together the yogurt, lemon juice and zest, mustard, garlic, and oregano. Stir into the chicken mixture.

3. Spoon into the pita pocket halves.

Time-saving tip: To quickly mince garlic, put the clove with the skin still on through a press. It will peel the garlic and mince it at the same time.

Per serving: *Calories: 199; Total Fat: 4g; Saturated Fat: 1g; Cholesterol: 59mg; Carbohydrates: 21g; Fiber: 3g; Protein: 22g*

TURKEY BACON, AVOCADO, AND TOMATO SANDWICHES

Serves 4 · **Prep time:** 15 minutes

The nice thing about this quick sandwich is you can make it spicy or mild depending on your own personal taste. As you mash the avocado with the other ingredients, taste it and add more hot sauce as desired to adjust the level of spiciness. This sandwich tastes best when tomatoes are in season.

1 avocado, pitted, peeled, and mashed

Juice of ½ lemon

1 garlic clove, minced

⅛ teaspoon sea salt

Dash hot sauce (optional)

8 slices whole-grain bread, toasted

8 slices peppered turkey bacon, cooked, drained, and cut in half

4 large tomato slices

1. In a small bowl, mash the avocado with the lemon juice, garlic, salt, and hot sauce (if using).

2. Spread on 4 slices of toast.

3. Top with the bacon slices and tomato. Top with the second piece of toast.

Technique tip: To remove the peel and pit from the avocado, hold it in one hand and carefully run a chef's knife around the edge of the avocado to halve it lengthwise. Then twist to separate the halves. Use a spoon to remove the pit, and then use a large spoon to scoop the flesh from the avocado skins. Always sprinkle avocado flesh with lemon juice as soon as you've removed it from its skin so it doesn't brown.

Per serving: *Calories: 361; Total Fat: 11g; Saturated Fat: 2g; Cholesterol: 40mg; Carbohydrates: 42g; Fiber: 8g; Protein: 22g*

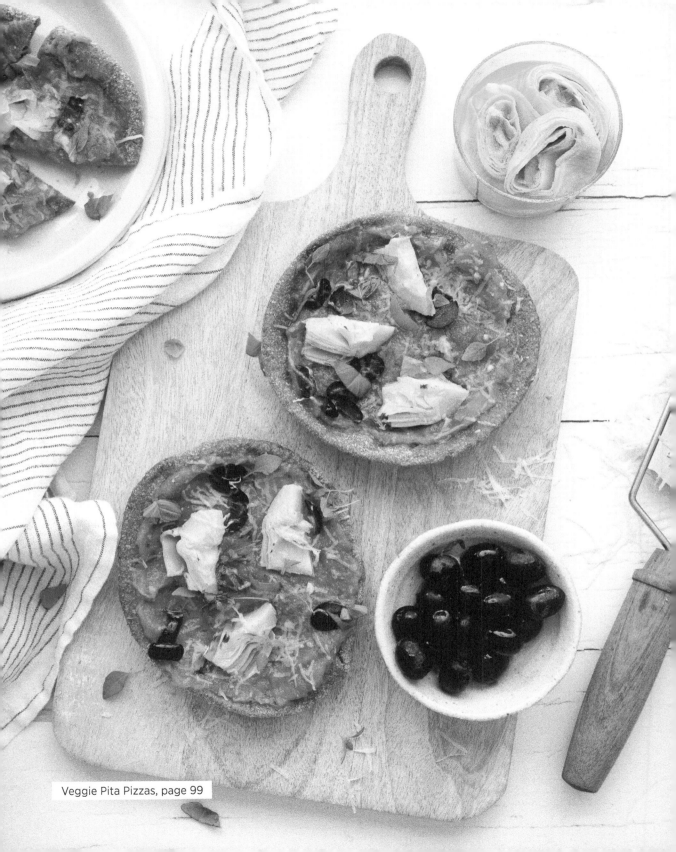

Veggie Pita Pizzas, page 99

Meatless Mains

Dairy-free, Gluten-free, Nut-free, Vegan

VEGAN CHILI

Serves 4 · **Prep time:** 10 minutes · **Cook time:** 30 minutes

Chili is the quintessential winter supper with its rich tomato sauce and warm chili spices. This version comes together quickly, and it freezes well so feel free to double the recipe and save it in the freezer in single-serving containers for quick reheating.

2 tablespoons
extra-virgin olive oil

1 yellow onion,
chopped

1 green bell pepper,
chopped

2 (15-ounce) cans
low-sodium kidney
beans, drained
and rinsed

2 (28-ounce) cans
crushed tomatoes

1 cup water

2 tablespoons chili
powder

1½ teaspoons
ground cumin

1 teaspoon
garlic powder

½ teaspoon sea salt

1. In a large pot, heat the olive oil on medium-high until it shimmers. Add the onion and bell pepper and cook for about 5 minutes, stirring occasionally, until the vegetables are soft.

2. Add the kidney beans, crushed tomatoes and their juices, water, chili powder, cumin, garlic powder, and salt.

3. Bring to a simmer, stirring occasionally. Reduce the heat to medium and simmer, stirring occasionally, for 15 minutes, until the flavors meld.

Variation tip: If you like your chili with some fire, then you can add up to ½ teaspoon of cayenne; add a little at a time, taste, and adjust for your desired heat level.

Per serving: *Calories: 402; Total Fat: 10g; Saturated Fat: 2g; Cholesterol: 0mg; Carbohydrates: 68g; Fiber: 18g; Protein: 19g*

WHOLE-WHEAT PASTA WITH WALNUT-KALE PESTO

Serves 4 · **Prep time:** 10 minutes · **Cook time:** 10 minutes

You can enjoy this pesto on whole-wheat noodles, or use it as a sauce or topping for roasted vegetables, baked sweet potatoes, and more. It's a versatile and simple pasta topping that's packed with plenty of flavor.

8 ounces whole-wheat pasta (any shape)

1 cup stemmed and chopped fresh kale

½ cup fresh basil leaves

¼ cup extra-virgin olive oil

¼ cup walnuts

Juice and zest of ½ lemon

3 garlic cloves, peeled

½ teaspoon sea salt

Pinch red pepper flakes

1. Bring a large pot of water to a boil and cook the pasta according to the package directions.

2. Meanwhile, in a blender or food processor, combine the kale, basil, olive oil, walnuts, lemon juice and zest, garlic, salt, and red pepper flakes. Pulse for 20 to 30 (1-second) pulses, until everything is well chopped.

3. Drain the pasta and toss with the pesto to serve.

Variation tip: Add cheesy flavor to this vegan pesto by adding 2 tablespoons of nutritional yeast. Make it nut-free by replacing the walnuts with pepitas (hulled pumpkin seeds).

Per serving: *Calories: 376; Total Fat: 20g; Saturated Fat: 3g; Cholesterol: 0mg; Carbohydrates: 45g; Fiber: 6g; Protein: 10g*

Dairy-free, Nut-free, Vegan

PASTA PRIMAVERA

Serves 4 · **Prep time:** 10 minutes · **Cook time:** 20 minutes

In-season, fresh veggies make this simple pasta dish bright, colorful, and packed with nutrition. Fresh herbs add color and bright flavors, which make this an aromatic meal that's a feast for the eyes, nose, and mouth.

8 ounces whole-wheat penne

2 tablespoons extra-virgin olive oil

2 bell peppers (red, orange, or yellow), cut into thin strips

2 medium summer squash (zucchini or yellow squash), halved lengthwise and sliced

1 red onion, halved and thinly sliced

4 garlic cloves, minced

1 pint cherry tomatoes, halved

Juice and zest of 1 lemon

½ teaspoon sea salt

10 fresh basil leaves, cut into strips

1. Bring a large pot of water to a boil and cook the pasta according to the package directions. Drain and set aside.

2. Meanwhile, in a large skillet or sauté pan, heat the olive oil on medium-high until it shimmers. Add the bell peppers, squash, and onion and cook for about 5 minutes, stirring occasionally, until the vegetables begin to soften.

3. Add the garlic and cook, stirring constantly, for 30 seconds, until fragrant.

4. Add the cherry tomatoes, lemon juice and zest, and salt. Cook, stirring, for another 5 minutes to soften the tomatoes.

5. Remove from the heat and stir in the basil. Toss with the pasta and serve.

Variation tip: Add some heat to this pasta by adding up to ½ teaspoon of red pepper flakes when you add the tomatoes.

Per serving: *Calories: 323; Total Fat: 9g; Saturated Fat: 1g; Cholesterol: 0mg; Carbohydrates: 55g; Fiber: 9g; Protein: 11g*

Dairy-free, Gluten-free, Nut-free, Vegan

MUSHROOM FAJITAS WITH GUACAMOLE

Serves 4 · **Prep time:** 15 minutes · **Cook time:** 20 minutes

Portobello mushrooms are a great choice for these fajitas because of their large size. However, if you're looking for a meatier texture, you can replace them with sliced shiitake mushrooms instead, which add a toothsome bite to these spicy fajitas.

8 soft corn tortillas

2 tablespoons
    extra-virgin olive oil

4 large portobello
    mushrooms, stems,
    gills removed,
    thinly sliced

1 red onion,
    thinly sliced

1 green bell pepper, cut
    into sticks

4 garlic cloves, minced

Juice of 1 lime

1 teaspoon
    chili powder

½ teaspoon sea salt

1 recipe Guacamole
    (page 150, omit the
    jicama), divided

1. Preheat the oven to 350°F.

2. Wrap the tortillas in aluminum foil and place them in the oven for 15 to 20 minutes to warm.

3. Meanwhile, in a large skillet or sauté pan, heat the olive oil on medium-high until it shimmers. Add the mushrooms, onion, and bell pepper. Cook for about 8 minutes, stirring occasionally, until the vegetables are soft and the mushrooms are browned.

4. Add the garlic and cook, stirring constantly, for 30 seconds, until fragrant.

5. Add the lime juice, chili powder, and salt. Cook, stirring, for 2 minutes more, until heated through.

6. Serve on the warmed tortillas with the guacamole on the side.

Technique tip: To prepare the portobellos, wipe them clean with a paper towel (don't rinse them, or they'll soak up a ton of water and become water-logged). Then use a sharp knife to remove the stem, and scrape away the gills with the edge of a spoon.

Per serving: *Calories: 328; Total Fat: 15g; Saturated Fat: 2g; Cholesterol: 0mg; Carbohydrates: 44g; Fiber: 5g; Protein: 10g*

BLACK BEAN-STUFFED SWEET POTATOES

Serves 4 · **Prep time:** 15 minutes · **Cook time:** 1 hour

Sweet potatoes have an earthy sweetness and serve as the perfect base for this simple black bean stuffing. Prepare the beans while the potatoes bake. If you're planning on taking this dish as a lunch, store the potatoes and beans separately and reheat in the microwave.

4 sweet potatoes, poked with a fork several times

2 tablespoons extra-virgin olive oil

1 red onion, thinly sliced

1 red bell pepper, chopped

1 (15-ounce) can black beans, drained and rinsed

1 teaspoon garlic powder

1 teaspoon ground cumin

½ teaspoon chipotle chili powder

½ teaspoon sea salt

¼ cup chopped fresh cilantro

1. Preheat the oven to 425°F.

2. Place the sweet potatoes on a rimmed baking sheet and bake for about 50 minutes, until they are soft.

3. Meanwhile, in a skillet or sauté pan, heat the olive oil on medium-high until it shimmers. Add the onion and bell pepper and cook for about 5 minutes, stirring occasionally, until soft.

4. Add the beans, garlic powder, cumin, chili powder, and salt. Cook, stirring occasionally, for 5 minutes more, until heated through.

5. Remove from the heat and stir in the cilantro.

6. Split the cooked potatoes and spoon the black bean filling into their centers to serve.

Substitution tip: If having beans and sweet potatoes feels like too much starch, replace the black beans with 8 ounces of chopped mushrooms.

Per serving: *Calories: 301; Total Fat: 8g; Saturated Fat: 1g; Cholesterol: 0mg; Carbohydrates: 51g; Fiber: 13g; Protein: 9g*

Dairy-free, Gluten-free, Nut-free, Vegan

CHICKPEA CURRY

Serves 4 · **Prep time:** 15 minutes · **Cook time:** 30 minutes

Using precooked brown rice (you'll find it in the grocery store rice aisle or freezer section) makes this curry quick and easy. Feel free to add more spices, such as cumin or coriander, to season the curry to your taste.

2 tablespoons extra-virgin olive oil

1 yellow onion, sliced

2 carrots, peeled and sliced

2 cups stemmed and chopped fresh kale

2 (15-ounce) cans chickpeas, drained and rinsed

1 (28-ounce) can crushed tomatoes

1 tablespoon curry powder

1 teaspoon garlic powder

½ teaspoon sea salt

2 cups cooked brown rice

1. In a large pot, heat the olive oil on medium-high until it shimmers. Add the onion, carrots, and kale and cook for about 5 minutes, stirring occasionally, until soft.

2. Add the chickpeas, tomatoes and their juices, curry powder, garlic powder, and salt. Bring to a simmer. Cook, stirring occasionally, for 10 minutes.

3. Spoon over the hot rice to serve.

Time-saving tip: You can also precook rice and save it in ½ cup portions in your freezer to save time and for use in recipes, because brown rice takes about 45 minutes to cook.

Per serving: *Calories: 472; Total Fat: 13g; Saturated Fat: 2g; Cholesterol: 0mg; Carbohydrates: 79g; Fiber: 17g; Protein: 17g*

Dairy-free, Gluten-free, Nut-free, Vegan

MEDITERRANEAN SPICED LENTILS AND QUINOA

Serves 4 • **Prep time:** 15 minutes • **Cook time:** 20 minutes

Warm and fragrant Mediterranean spices make these simple lentils something special. This freezes well, so make extra and store it in the freezer for up to 6 months.

1½ cups water

¾ cup quinoa, rinsed

2 tablespoons extra-virgin olive oil

1 yellow onion, chopped

2 (15-ounce) cans lentils, drained

1 (15-ounce) can crushed tomatoes

1 teaspoon ground cumin

1 teaspoon dried oregano

½ teaspoon ground coriander

½ teaspoon ground cinnamon

½ teaspoon sea salt

1. In a large saucepan, combine the water and quinoa. Bring to a boil on medium-high heat. Then reduce the heat to medium-low, cover, and cook for 15 minutes. Let stand, covered, for 5 minutes off the heat, then remove the cover and fluff with a fork.

2. Meanwhile, in a large skillet or sauté pan, heat the olive oil on medium-high until it shimmers.

3. Add the onion and cook for about 5 minutes, stirring occasionally, until soft.

4. Add the lentils, crushed tomatoes and their juices, cumin, oregano, coriander, cinnamon, and salt. Bring to a simmer, stirring. Continue to cook for 5 to 7 minutes, stirring occasionally, until the mixture thickens.

5. Spoon over the hot quinoa to serve.

Technique tip: Quinoa can have a bitter flavor if it's not well rinsed. Place the dry quinoa in a wire-mesh sieve and run it under cold water, rubbing it with your fingertips, to remove the saponin that coats it and creates the bitter flavor.

Per serving: *Calories: 437; Total Fat: 10g; Saturated Fat: 1g; Cholesterol: 0mg; Carbohydrates: 69g; Fiber: 16g; Protein: 22g*

Dairy-free, Nut-free, Vegan

TOFU AND VEGETABLE STIR-FRY

Serves 4 · **Prep time:** 15 minutes · **Cook time:** 15 minutes

Serve this Asian-inspired tofu stir-fry over cooked brown rice or cooked quinoa for a delicious meatless main. You can save time by purchasing lightly dried ginger, which is available in the produce section of the grocery store.

2 tablespoons extra-virgin olive oil

2 cups broccoli florets

1 red bell pepper, sliced

1 bunch scallions, both white and green parts, thinly sliced

12 ounces extra-firm tofu, chopped

5 garlic cloves, sliced

1 tablespoon peeled and grated fresh ginger

1 tablespoon low-sodium soy sauce or tamari

½ teaspoon sesame oil

Juice of 1 lime

1. In a large skillet or sauté pan, heat the olive oil on medium-high until it shimmers. Add the broccoli, bell pepper, and scallions and cook for 3 to 5 minutes, stirring occasionally, until veggies are crisp-tender.

2. Add the tofu, garlic, and ginger and cook for another 5 minutes, stirring, until heated through.

3. Add the soy sauce, sesame oil, and lime juice. Cook, stirring, for 2 minutes more, until the flavors meld.

Technique tip: Before using the tofu, remove some of the water from it so it gets a good sear. To do this, place the tofu in a colander in the sink and place a plate on top of it. Put a few cans or something heavy to weigh the tofu down and let it drain for about 30 minutes before chopping.

Per serving: *Calories: 197; Total Fat: 12g; Saturated Fat: 2g; Cholesterol: 0mg; Carbohydrates: 12g; Fiber: 4g; Protein: 11g*

Dairy-free, Vegetarian

ALMOND BUTTER NOODLES

Serves 4 · **Prep time:** 15 minutes · **Cook time:** 10 minutes

Inspired by the flavors of Thai peanut sauce, these delicious noodles are fast and easy, and they keep exceptionally well. They are also delicious cold or hot, so they make a great meal on the go.

8 ounces whole-wheat angel hair pasta

¼ cup almond butter

2 tablespoons rice vinegar

1 tablespoon sesame oil

1 tablespoon low-sodium soy sauce or tamari

1 tablespoon honey

1 garlic clove, peeled

1 teaspoon peeled and grated fresh ginger

2 scallions, both white and green parts, thinly sliced

2 teaspoons sesame seeds

1. Bring a large pot of water to a boil and cook the pasta according to the package directions.

2. Meanwhile, in a blender or food processor, combine the almond butter, vinegar, sesame oil, soy sauce, honey, garlic, and ginger. Blend until smooth.

3. Drain the pasta and toss with the sauce. Garnish with the scallions and sesame seeds to serve.

Variation tip: Looking for some additional crunch? Garnish with 2 tablespoons of chopped almonds.

Per serving: *Calories: 360; Total Fat: 15g; Saturated Fat: 2g; Cholesterol: 0mg; Carbohydrates: 50g; Fiber: 7g; Protein: 12g*

Nut-free, Vegetarian

VEGGIE PITA PIZZAS

Serves 4 · **Prep time:** 15 minutes · **Cook time:** 10 minutes

Pizza night just got easier and healthier. Whole-wheat pitas make a great fast pizza crust. You can even lay out vegetables and let the family top their own pizzas for a fun, interactive family dinner.

4 whole-wheat pita rounds

1 (15-ounce) can chopped tomatoes with garlic and basil, drained

1 teaspoon dried Italian herbs

¼ teaspoon sea salt

1 cup jarred roasted red peppers, drained, rinsed, and chopped

1 cup water-packed artichoke hearts, drained, rinsed, and chopped

½ red onion, chopped

1 (2-ounce) can sliced black olives, rinsed and drained

½ cup shredded Parmesan cheese

10 fresh basil leaves, cut into strips

1. Preheat the oven to 425°F.

2. Place the whole pitas on a rimmed baking sheet.

3. In a blender or food processor, combine the tomatoes, Italian herbs, and salt. Blend until smooth. Transfer to a small saucepan and heat on medium-high until it simmers, stirring occasionally. Spread on the pita rounds.

4. Sprinkle the pitas with the roasted peppers, artichoke hearts, onion, and olives. Sprinkle with the cheese.

5. Bake for 8 to 10 minutes, until the cheese is melted and browned.

6. Garnish with the basil and serve.

Time-saving tip: You can also use commercially prepared flatbreads or whole-wheat tortillas in place of the pitas as your pizza crust.

Per serving: Calories: 280; Total Fat: 6g; Saturated Fat: 2g; Cholesterol: 10mg; Carbohydrates: 47g; Fiber: 8g; Protein: 14g

Dairy-free, Vegan

PASTA WITH ROMESCO SAUCE

Serves 4 • **Prep time:** 5 minutes • **Cook time:** 12 minutes

Romesco sauce is a bright, flavorful, simple no-cook sauce that's easy to make. While this recipe calls for you to toss it with pasta, it's also good as a vegetable topping, pizza sauce, or on a baked potato or sweet potato.

8 ounces whole-wheat pasta (any shape)

1 pint cherry tomatoes

1 (12-ounce) jar roasted red peppers, rinsed and drained

½ cup raw almonds

¼ cup fresh Italian parsley

Juice of 1 lemon

2 tablespoons extra-virgin olive oil

3 garlic cloves, peeled

½ teaspoon sea salt

1. Bring a large pot of water to a boil and cook the pasta according to the package directions.

2. Meanwhile, in a blender or food processor, combine the cherry tomatoes, roasted red peppers, almonds, parsley, lemon juice, olive oil, garlic, and salt. Blend until smooth.

3. Drain the pasta and toss with the sauce to serve.

Technique tip: It's easy to make your own roasted red peppers; simply slice the peppers (removing the ribs and seeds), put them on a rimmed baking sheet, brush with a little olive oil, and cook in a 400°F oven until soft and lightly charred, about 20 minutes.

Per serving: *Calories: 393; Total Fat: 17g; Saturated Fat:2 g; Cholesterol: 0mg; Carbohydrates: 53g; Fiber: 9g; Protein: 13g*

SPAGHETTI SQUASH MARINARA

Serves 4 · **Prep time:** 10 minutes · **Cook time:** 40 minutes

Most of the cook time for this recipe is inactive time while you wait for the spaghetti squash to bake. It makes an excellent stand-in for noodles in this simple yet delicious recipe.

1 large spaghetti squash, halved and seeded

4 tablespoons extra-virgin olive oil, divided

1 yellow onion, chopped

1 red bell pepper, chopped

4 garlic cloves, minced

1 (28-ounce) can crushed tomatoes

1 tablespoon dried Italian herbs

½ teaspoon sea salt

Pinch red pepper flakes

1. Preheat the oven to 400°F.

2. Brush the flesh side of the spaghetti squash with 2 tablespoons of olive oil and place, cut-side down, on a rimmed baking sheet. Bake for 40 minutes, until soft and easily pierced with a fork.

3. Meanwhile, in a large pot, heat the remaining 2 tablespoons of olive oil on medium-high until it shimmers. Add the onion and bell pepper and cook for 5 minutes, stirring occasionally, until soft.

4. Add the garlic and cook, stirring constantly, for 30 seconds, until fragrant.

5. Add the tomatoes and their juices, Italian herbs, salt, and red pepper flakes. Bring to a simmer. Cook, stirring occasionally, for 10 minutes.

6. When the squash is cooked, remove it from the oven and turn it cut-side up. Use a fork to scrape the squash into noodles.

7. Serve the squash topped with the marinara sauce.

Per serving: Calories: 265; Total Fat: 15g; Saturated Fat: 2g; Cholesterol: 0mg; Carbohydrates: 34g; Fiber: 8g; Protein: 6g

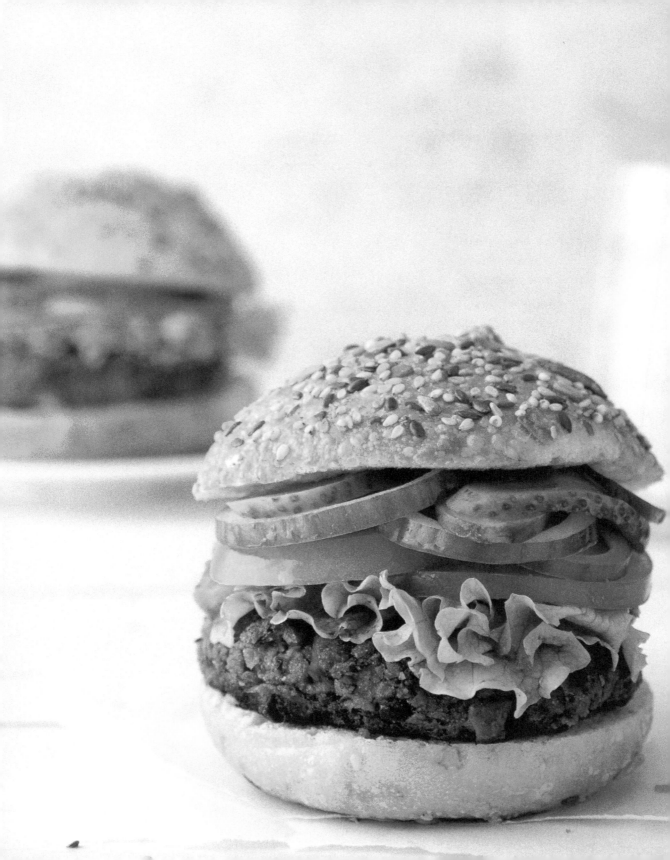

Dairy-free, Nut-free, Vegetarian

BLACK BEAN BURGERS

Serves 4 · **Prep time:** 10 minutes · **Cook time:** 40 minutes

There are all kinds of ways you can serve these black bean patties. Serve them on whole-grain buns with all the fixings to make a burger, or wrap them in lettuce for a tasty wrap. You can even eat the burgers by themselves, topped with romesco sauce, guacamole, or pesto.

2 bell peppers (any color), chopped

1 red onion, chopped

2 tablespoons extra-virgin olive oil

1 (15-ounce) can black beans, drained and rinsed

½ cup whole-wheat bread crumbs

2 large eggs, beaten

1 teaspoon sea salt

1 teaspoon garlic powder

1 teaspoon chili powder

½ teaspoon chipotle chili powder

1. Preheat the oven to 375°F. Line a rimmed baking sheet with parchment paper.

2. In a blender or food processor, pulse the bell peppers and red onion until they are very finely chopped, about 15 (1-second) pulses.

3. In a skillet or sauté pan, heat the olive oil on medium-high. Add the bell pepper and onion and cook, stirring occasionally, for 5 minutes. Let cool and return to the food processor or blender.

4. Add the black beans, bread crumbs, eggs, salt, garlic powder, chili powder, and chipotle chili powder. Pulse for 20 (1-second) pulses, or until well mixed.

5. Form into 4 patties and place on the prepared baking sheet. Bake for 20 minutes. Flip and bake for another 20 minutes.

Substitution tip: Substitute an equal amount of any cooked, canned, and drained beans such as kidney beans or chickpeas.

Per serving: *Calories: 282; Total Fat: 11g; Saturated Fat: 2g; Cholesterol: 93mg; Carbohydrates: 37g; Fiber: 11g; Protein: 12g*

VEGGIE AND BROWN RICE-STUFFED BELL PEPPERS

Serves 4 · **Prep time:** 10 minutes · **Cook time:** 40 minutes

While these take about 40 minutes to bake, they don't take long to prepare. Use precooked brown rice (or an equal amount of precooked quinoa) to save time.

4 bell peppers (any color), tops cut off and chopped, ribs and seeds removed

2 tablespoons extra-virgin olive oil

8 ounces cremini mushrooms, chopped

2 medium summer squash (zucchini, pattypan, yellow), chopped

1 yellow onion, chopped

4 garlic cloves, minced

1 (14.5-ounce) can crushed tomatoes, drained

1 cup cooked brown rice

1 teaspoon dried thyme

½ teaspoon sea salt

1. Preheat the oven to 375°F.

2. Place the peppers, cut-side up, in a baking dish.

3. In a large skillet or sauté pan, heat the olive oil on medium-high. Add the mushrooms, squash, onion, and chopped pepper tops. Cook for about 5 minutes, stirring occasionally, until the vegetables are soft.

4. Add the garlic and cook, stirring constantly, for 30 seconds, until fragrant. Add the tomatoes, rice, thyme, and salt. Cook, stirring occasionally, for 5 minutes more, until heated through. Spoon into the prepared peppers.

5. Bake, covered with aluminum foil, for about 40 minutes, until the peppers are soft.

Technique tip: Don't waste the pepper tops. Cut any usable vegetable away from the stems and then chop the tops and add them to the vegetables when you cook the onions.

Per serving: *Calories: 232; Total Fat: 8g; Saturated Fat: 1g; Cholesterol: 0mg; Carbohydrates: 37g; Fiber: 7g; Protein: 7g*

Dairy-free, Gluten-free, Nut-free, Vegan

CAJUN-INSPIRED RED BEANS AND RICE

Serves 4 · **Prep time:** 15 minutes · **Cook time:** 20 minutes

One of the foundations of Cajun and Creole cooking is the use of a mix of ingredients called the Holy Trinity: onions, bell peppers, and celery. These three ingredients serve as the flavor foundation of most Cajun food, including this simple red beans and rice dish.

2 tablespoons extra-virgin olive oil

1 yellow onion, finely chopped

1 green bell pepper, finely chopped

2 celery stalks, finely chopped

4 garlic cloves, minced

2 (15-ounce) cans kidney beans, drained and rinsed

2 teaspoons Cajun seasoning blend

1 teaspoon dried thyme

½ teaspoon sea salt

2 cups cooked brown rice, hot

1. In a large skillet or sauté pan, heat the olive oil on medium-high. Add the onions, bell pepper, and celery and cook for 5 minutes, stirring frequently, until softened.

2. Add the garlic and cook, stirring constantly, for 30 seconds, until fragrant.

3. Add the kidney beans, Cajun seasoning, thyme, and salt. Cook, stirring, for 5 minutes, until heated through.

4. Add the rice and cook, stirring, for 3 minutes more.

Substitution tip: Make your own Cajun seasoning with ½ teaspoon of smoked paprika, ¼ teaspoon of garlic powder, ¼ teaspoon of dried oregano, ¼ teaspoon of cayenne, ¼ teaspoon of onion powder, and ¼ teaspoon of black pepper.

Per serving: *Calories: 405; Total Fat: 10g; Saturated Fat: 2g; Cholesterol: 0mg; Carbohydrates: 66g; Fiber: 12g; Protein: 16g*

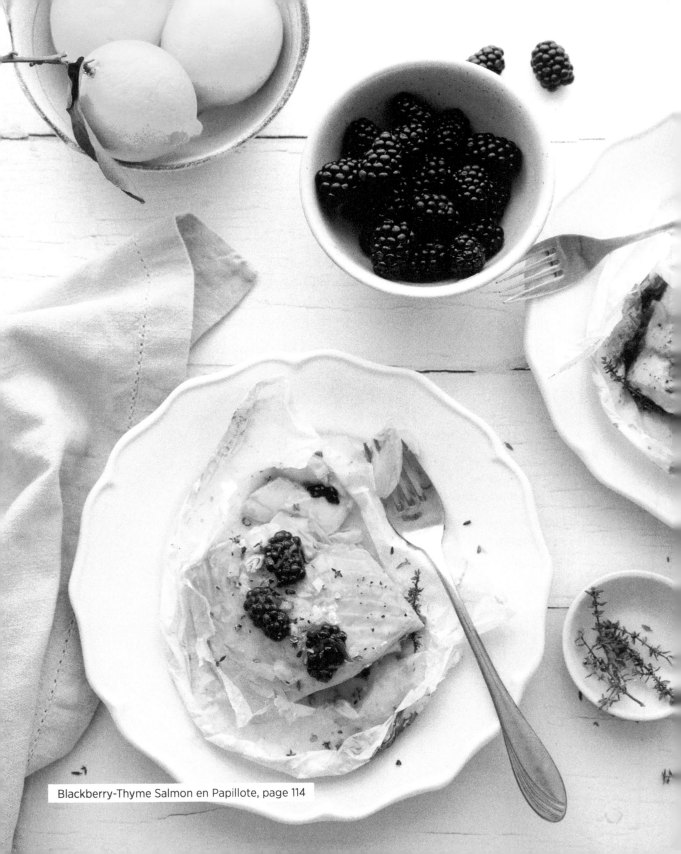
Blackberry-Thyme Salmon en Papillote, page 114

Seafood & Poultry Mains

Dairy-free, Gluten-free, Nut-free

SHRIMP SCAMPI WITH ZOODLES

Serves 4 · **Prep time:** 15 minutes · **Cook time:** 15 minutes

Zoodles (zucchini noodles) lighten up this Italian-inspired shrimp scampi recipe, which is fragrant with garlic, lemon, and herbs. Save time by buying shrimp that has already been peeled and deveined, with tails removed.

3 medium zucchini

2 tablespoons extra-virgin olive oil

1 shallot, minced

1 pound medium shrimp, peeled, deveined, and tails cut off

4 garlic cloves, minced

Juice of 3 lemons and zest of 1, divided

½ teaspoon sea salt

¼ teaspoon freshly ground black pepper

Pinch red pepper flakes

¼ cup chopped fresh Italian parsley

1. Using a vegetable peeler, cut the zucchini into long strips. Use a sharp knife to cut each strip in half lengthwise to create ribbons. Set aside.

2. In a large skillet or sauté pan, heat the olive oil on medium-high until it shimmers. Add the shallot and cook for 3 to 5 minutes, stirring frequently, until soft.

3. Add the shrimp and cook for 3 to 5 minutes, stirring occasionally, until the shrimp is pink.

4. Add the garlic and cook, stirring constantly, for 30 seconds, until fragrant.

5. Add the lemon juice, salt, black pepper, red pepper flakes, and zucchini. Cook, stirring, for 5 minutes more.

6. Remove from the heat and stir in the parsley and lemon zest.

Technique tip: To devein shrimp, after removing the peel and tail, use a sharp knife and slit along the back of the shrimp. Use the tip of the knife to remove the vein, and then rinse the cleaned shrimp under cool running water. Drain in a colander.

Per serving: *Calories: 186; Total Fat: 8g; Saturated Fat: 1g; Cholesterol: 155mg; Carbohydrates: 10g; Fiber: 2g; Protein: 20g*

Dairy-free, Gluten-free, Nut-free

ORANGE-SCENTED POACHED COD WITH BELL PEPPERS

Serves 4 · **Prep time:** 10 minutes · **Cook time:** 15 minutes

Cod cooks very quickly, so this is a quick, easy, and nutritious recipe with lots of flavor. You can use any bell peppers: red, yellow, orange, purple, or a combination thereof for a colorful presentation.

2 tablespoons extra-virgin olive oil

2 bell peppers (any color), thinly sliced

1 sweet onion, halved and thinly sliced

½ cup freshly squeezed orange juice

½ teaspoon sea salt

⅛ teaspoon freshly ground black pepper

1 teaspoon dried tarragon

4 (4-ounce) cod fillets, pin bones removed

1. In a large skillet or sauté pan with a lid, heat the olive oil on medium-high until it shimmers. Add the bell pepper and onion and cook for about 5 minutes, stirring occasionally, until soft.

2. Add the orange juice, salt, black pepper, and tarragon. Bring to a simmer.

3. Add the cod. Cover and steam for about 8 minutes, until the fish is opaque and flaky.

Substitution tip: Change the flavor profile of this dish by replacing the fresh orange juice and tarragon with equal amounts of fresh lemon juice and dried dill.

Per serving: *Calories: 188; Total Fat: 8g; Saturated Fat: 1g; Cholesterol: 59mg; Carbohydrates: 10g; Fiber: 2g; Protein: 21g*

Dairy-free, Gluten-free, Nut-free

HERBED HALIBUT AND SUMMER SQUASH IN PARCHMENT

Serves 4 · **Prep time:** 10 minutes · **Cook time:** 15 minutes

Halibut is a mild, sweet white fish that maintains its tenderness when it's steamed in parchment in the oven. You can also replace the halibut with any other white-fleshed fish if halibut isn't readily available.

4 (4-ounce) halibut fillets

½ teaspoon sea salt

⅛ teaspoon freshly ground black pepper

3 tablespoons chopped fresh dill

Zest of 1 lemon and juice of 3 lemons, divided

2 medium summer squash (zucchini, pattypan, yellow), sliced into ¼-inch-thick rounds

1 shallot, thinly sliced

2 tablespoons extra-virgin olive oil

1. Preheat the oven to 375°F.

2. Place 4 (12-inch) square pieces of parchment paper on a rimmed baking sheet. Place a halibut fillet on each parchment piece, and season with the salt, pepper, dill, and lemon zest.

3. Fold into packets, leaving the top open. Add the squash and shallot.

4. Drizzle with the olive oil and lemon juice and seal the packets at the top.

5. Bake for about 15 minutes, until the vegetables are tender, and the fish is opaque and flaky.

Technique tip: Make sure you've removed any small bones from the fish before using it. In a well-lit place, examine the fish and use pliers or tweezers to remove any bones.

Per serving: *Calories: 195; Total Fat: 9g; Saturated Fat: 1g; Cholesterol: 56mg; Carbohydrates: 7g; Fiber: 1g; Protein: 23g*

Dairy-free, Gluten-free, Nut-free

GRILLED FISH TACOS

Serves 4 · **Prep time:** 10 minutes · **Cook time:** 15 minutes

You can use any type of grill for these tacos: a grill pan, an indoor grill such as a George Foreman grill, or an outdoor gas or charcoal grill. You'll need to oil the grill well with olive oil to keep it from sticking.

Juice of 3 limes

¼ cup extra-virgin olive oil, plus extra for oiling the grill

¼ cup fresh cilantro

3 scallions, both white and green parts, chopped

3 garlic cloves, minced

1 teaspoon chili powder

½ teaspoon sea salt

1 pound boneless, skinless white fish, such as cod

8 soft corn tortillas

½ cup jarred salsa

1. In a blender or food processor, combine the lime juice, olive oil, cilantro, scallions, garlic, chili powder, and salt. Pulse for 15 (1-second) pulses. Pour all but 2 tablespoons of the marinade into a shallow dish. Add the cod. Allow to sit for 5 minutes in the marinade, then turn it and marinate on the other side for another 5 minutes.

2. Preheat the oven to 350°F.

3. Wrap the tortillas in aluminum foil and heat for about 10 minutes, until warmed.

4. Preheat the grill on medium-high and oil it.

5. Pat the cod dry, removing the marinade with a paper towel. Grill for about 5 minutes per side, until opaque and flaky.

6. Remove the cod from the grill and cut it into pieces. Put it in a bowl and stir in the reserved marinade.

7. Wrap in the warm tortillas and serve with the salsa.

Per serving: *Calories: 333; Total Fat: 15g; Saturated Fat: 2g; Cholesterol: 59mg; Carbohydrates: 28g; Fiber: 3g; Protein: 23g*

Dairy-free, Gluten-free, Nut-free

TILAPIA WITH MANGO SALSA

Serves 4 · **Prep time:** 10 minutes · **Cook time:** 12 minutes

Prepare the simple but flavorful salsa while the tilapia cooks in the oven; you'll have dinner on the table in less than 15 minutes. If you can't find fresh tilapia, it's usually available in the seafood freezer section at the grocery store.

4 (4-ounce) tilapia fillets

1 tablespoon extra-virgin olive oil

¾ teaspoon sea salt, divided

¼ teaspoon freshly ground black pepper

2 mangos, peeled, pitted, and cubed

½ red onion, finely chopped

1 jalapeño pepper, ribs and seeds removed, finely chopped

2 tablespoons chopped fresh cilantro

Juice of 1 lime

1. Preheat the oven to 400°F.

2. Place the fish on a rimmed baking sheet. Brush with the olive oil and season with ½ teaspoon of salt and the pepper.

3. Bake for 10 to 12 minutes, until the fish is opaque and flaky.

4. Meanwhile, in a small bowl, combine the mango, onion, jalapeño, cilantro, lime juice, and remaining ¼ teaspoon of salt. Mix well.

5. Serve the fish with the salsa spooned over the top.

Time-saving tip: Save time by purchasing precut mango in the produce section of the grocery store, or you can use frozen mango that has been thawed.

Per serving: *Calories: 249; Total Fat: 6g; Saturated Fat: 1g; Cholesterol: 57mg; Carbohydrates: 28g; Fiber: 3g; Protein: 24g*

ORANGE-MAPLE-GINGER SALMON

Serves 4 · **Prep time:** 5 minutes · **Cook time:** 15 minutes

Serve this salmon with a simple salad or a veggie side dish for a flavorful, fast meal. Because fish is so delicate, it marinates very quickly—only about 5 minutes while the oven preheats is perfect.

¼ **cup freshly squeezed orange juice**

2 **tablespoons pure maple syrup**

2 **tablespoons peeled and grated fresh ginger**

1 **tablespoon low-sodium soy sauce or tamari**

½ **teaspoon Dijon mustard**

4 **(4-ounce) salmon fillets**

1. Preheat the oven to 450°F.

2. In a shallow dish, whisk together the orange juice, maple syrup, ginger, soy sauce, and mustard.

3. Place the salmon, flesh-side down, in the marinade and allow to sit for 5 to 10 minutes.

4. Remove the salmon from the marinade and pat dry. Place on a rimmed baking sheet, skin-side down.

5. Bake for about 15 minutes, until the salmon is opaque and flaky and reaches an internal temperature of 145°F.

Substitution tip: For an Asian-inspired flavor profile, replace the orange juice and maple syrup with equal amounts of fresh lime juice and honey and add ½ teaspoon of sesame oil. Garnish with thinly sliced scallions and 1 tablespoon of sesame seeds.

Per serving: *Calories: 161; Total Fat: 3g; Saturated Fat: 1g; Cholesterol: 64mg; Carbohydrates: 10g; Fiber: <1g; Protein: 22g*

BLACKBERRY-THYME SALMON EN PAPILLOTE

Serves 4 · **Prep time:** 5 minutes · **Cook time:** 25 minutes

En papillote is a French term that means cooked in a paper wrapper. Using parchment is a great way to cook all kinds of fish because it steams it and keeps it moist. To serve, simply open the paper packets at the top and place on a plate, still in the paper.

4 (4-ounce) salmon fillets

½ teaspoon sea salt

⅛ teaspoon freshly ground black pepper

1 cup fresh blackberries

Juice of 2 lemons

2 tablespoons minced shallot

1 teaspoon dried thyme

1. Preheat the oven to 400°F.

2. Place 4 (12-inch) square pieces of parchment paper on a rimmed baking sheet. Place a salmon fillet on each piece of parchment and sprinkle with salt and pepper. Fold the paper around the salmon into packets, leaving the top open with room to seal it.

3. In a small bowl, mix together the blackberries, lemon juice, shallot, and thyme. Divide evenly among the packets directly on top of the salmon.

4. Seal each packet and place the packets in the oven. Cook for about 25 minutes, until the salmon reaches an internal temperature of 145°F and is flaky.

Substitution tip: If it's easier, you can replace the parchment with aluminum foil, although the presentation won't be quite as pretty.

Per serving: *Calories: 155; Total Fat: 5g; Saturated Fat: 2g; Cholesterol: 55mg; Carbohydrates: 6g; Fiber: 2g; Protein: 23g*

Dairy-free

BAKED ALMOND-CRUSTED FISH STICKS

Serves 4 · **Prep time:** 10 minutes · **Cook time:** 15 minutes

Fish sticks are a family favorite, and this baked (not fried) version lightens up the classic frozen fish sticks that are so popular. Serve with a simple slaw, such as the Sweet and Spicy Slaw (page 71).

1 pound white-fleshed fish, such as cod, skin and bones removed

½ cup unsweetened plain almond milk or nondairy milk of choice

1 large egg, beaten

1 teaspoon Dijon mustard

½ cup almond flour

½ cup whole-wheat bread crumbs

1 teaspoon dried thyme

1 teaspoon garlic powder

1 teaspoon sea salt

¼ teaspoon freshly ground black pepper

1. Preheat the oven to 400°F. Line a rimmed baking sheet with parchment paper.

2. Cut the fish into 1-inch-wide-by-2-inch-long pieces.

3. In a medium bowl, whisk together the milk, egg, and mustard.

4. In shallow dish, whisk together the almond flour, bread crumbs, thyme, garlic powder, salt, and pepper.

5. Dip the cod pieces in the milk mixture and then in the bread crumb mixture, tapping off any excess coating. Place on the prepared baking sheet.

6. Bake for about 12 minutes, until the coating is golden and the fish is opaque.

Serving tip: Whisk up an easy tartar sauce for dipping: Combine ¼ cup of nonfat plain Greek yogurt, the zest and juice of ½ lemon, a finely chopped dill pickle, 1 tablespoon of chopped fresh dill, and ¼ teaspoon of cream of tartar.

Per serving: *Calories: 242; Total Fat: 10g; Saturated Fat: 1g; Cholesterol: 106mg; Carbohydrates: 14g; Fiber: 3g; Protein: 27g*

Dairy-free, Nut-free

TURKEY PICCATA

Serves 4 · **Prep time:** 5 minutes · **Cook time:** 10 minutes

Because the turkey cutlets are pounded thin, they cook quickly, so this is a fast recipe that can be on the table in less than 15 minutes.

½ cup whole-wheat flour

½ teaspoon sea salt

¼ teaspoon freshly ground black pepper

4 (3-ounce) turkey cutlets, pounded to ½-inch thickness

2 tablespoons extra-virgin olive oil

2 tablespoons minced shallot

1 garlic clove, sliced

½ cup low-sodium chicken broth

Juice of 2 lemons

1 tablespoon capers, drained and rinsed

1. In a flat dish, whisk together the flour, salt, and pepper.

2. Dip the turkey into the flour mixture and pat off any excess.

3. In a large, nonstick skillet or sauté pan, heat the olive oil on medium-high until it shimmers. Add the turkey pieces (you may need to work in batches so you don't overcrowd the pan—if you do, use ½ tablespoon of olive oil for each piece of turkey) and cook until the turkey is browned on both sides. Set aside on a platter.

4. Add the shallot and garlic to the pan and cook, stirring, for 1 minute.

5. Add the chicken broth, lemon juice, and capers and, using the side of a spoon, scrape any browned bits from the bottom of the pan. Bring to a simmer and cook for about 4 minutes, until the liquid is reduced by half.

6. Return the turkey pieces to the sauce and turn to coat. Serve with the sauce spooned on top.

Technique tip: To pound the turkey cutlets, place them between two pieces of plastic wrap or parchment and pound with a mallet or the side of a can.

Per serving: *Calories: 216; Total Fat: 8g; Saturated Fat: 1g; Cholesterol: 53mg; Carbohydrates: 14g; Fiber: 2g; Protein: 24g*

Dairy-free, Gluten-free, Nut-free

CRANBERRY AND SPINACH-STUFFED TURKEY BREAST

Serves 4 · **Prep time:** 10 minutes · **Cook time:** 50 minutes

Use turkey breast cutlets to make these simple stuffed turkey breast pieces. Pound each cutlet to ½-inch thickness (see Tip on page 116) so it's easy to wrap the stuffing. These will freeze well, so if you have more than 4 cutlets, you can make extra and freeze them.

4 (3-ounce) turkey breast cutlets, pounded to ½-inch thickness

1 teaspoon sea salt, divided

¼ teaspoon freshly ground black pepper

2 tablespoons extra-virgin olive oil

1 shallot, minced

8 cups fresh baby spinach

1 garlic clove, sliced

1 teaspoon dried sage

½ cup dried cranberries

1. Preheat the oven to 375°F. Line a rimmed baking sheet with parchment paper.

2. Season the turkey cutlets with ½ teaspoon of salt and the pepper and set aside.

3. In a large skillet or sauté pan, heat the olive oil on medium-high until it shimmers. Add the shallot and cook for about 3 minutes, stirring occasionally, until soft.

4. Add the spinach, garlic, and sage and cook for about 3 minutes more, stirring, until the spinach softens. Let cool.

5. Spoon the mixture on the prepared turkey and sprinkle with the cranberries. Roll lengthwise and tie with kitchen twine.

6. Bake for about 40 minutes, until the juices run clear.

Substitution tip: You can also use chicken breast halves in place of the turkey if you are unable to find turkey breast cutlets.

Per serving: *Calories: 234; Total Fat: 8g; Saturated Fat: 1g; Cholesterol: 53mg; Carbohydrates: 21g; Fiber: 3g; Protein: 23g*

Dairy-free, Nut-free

GROUND TURKEY STIR-FRY

Serves 4 · **Prep time:** 15 minutes · **Cook time:** 15 minutes

Stir-fries are super easy and quick, especially when you're using ground meat such as turkey. Keep fat and calories low by using the leanest turkey breast.

2 tablespoons extra-virgin olive oil

1 pound ground turkey breast

1 (10-ounce) bag tri-color coleslaw mix

1 bunch scallions, both white and green parts, thinly sliced

3 garlic cloves, sliced

1 tablespoon peeled and grated fresh ginger

Juice of 2 limes

1 tablespoon low-sodium soy sauce or tamari

½ teaspoon sesame oil

½ teaspoon sriracha (optional)

1. In a large skillet or sauté pan, heat the olive oil on medium-high until it shimmers. Add the turkey and cook for about 7 minutes, crumbling with a spoon, until it is browned.

2. Add the coleslaw mix, scallions, garlic, and ginger. Cook, stirring, until the vegetables soften, about 3 minutes more.

3. In a small bowl, whisk together the lime juice, soy sauce, sesame oil, and sriracha (if using). Add to the pan. Cook, stirring, for 2 minutes more, until heated through.

Substitution tip: You can also use a head of green cabbage in place of the tri-color coleslaw mix. To shred the cabbage, grate it on a box grater.

Per serving: Calories: 225; Total Fat: 8g; Saturated Fat: 1g; Cholesterol: 51mg; Carbohydrates: 10g; Fiber: 3g; Protein: 28g

Dairy-free, Gluten-free, Nut-free

ROASTED CHICKEN THIGHS AND ROOT VEGETABLES

Serves 4 · **Prep time:** 15 minutes · **Cook time:** 1 hour

This simple chicken and veggie bake doesn't take much active time, and with only one pan, you can minimize cleanup as well. It's a delicious full meal that will satisfy your entire family with Sunday dinner flavors.

10 ounces Brussels sprouts, halved and trimmed

10 ounces baby carrots

6 shallots, peeled and quartered

1 fennel bulb, cored and chopped

2 tablespoons extra-virgin olive oil

4 bone-in, skin-on chicken thighs

1 teaspoon dried thyme

½ teaspoon sea salt

¼ teaspoon freshly ground black pepper

1. Preheat the oven to 475°F.

2. In a large bowl, toss the Brussels sprouts, carrots, shallots, and fennel with the olive oil. Spread in a single layer on a large rimmed baking sheet.

3. Place the chicken on top of the vegetables and season with the thyme, salt, and pepper.

4. Roast for about 1 hour, until the chicken reaches an internal temperature of 165°F and the juices run clear.

Substitution tip: You can also use chicken drumsticks for this recipe. If you double the recipe for more people, you'll need 2 large rimmed baking sheets.

Per serving: *Calories: 417; Total Fat: 26g; Saturated Fat: 6g; Cholesterol: 110mg; Carbohydrates: 27g; Fiber: 9g; Protein: 24g*

Dairy-free, Nut-free

TERIYAKI CHICKEN SKEWERS

Serves 4 · **Prep time:** 10 minutes · **Cook time:** 25 minutes

It isn't hard to make homemade teriyaki sauce, and you can control the amount of salt and sugar if you make it yourself instead of using a commercially prepared brand. It's a delicious accompaniment to chicken breast skewers.

½ cup water

¼ cup honey or pure maple syrup

2 tablespoons low-sodium soy sauce

1 tablespoon peeled and grated fresh ginger

1 tablespoon cornstarch or arrowroot powder

¼ teaspoon garlic powder

1 pound boneless, skinless chicken breast, cut into 1-inch pieces

2 cups fresh pineapple, cut into 1-inch chunks

Olive oil, for greasing the grill

1. Preheat a grill or grill pan to medium-high.

2. In a small saucepan, whisk together the water, honey, soy sauce, ginger, cornstarch, and garlic powder. Bring to a simmer on medium-high. Simmer for about 5 minutes, whisking, until thick. Let cool and divide into two equal portions.

3. Thread the chicken and pineapple chunks onto skewers in alternating pieces.

4. Oil the grill and place the skewers on. As the skewers cook, brush them with one half of the teriyaki sauce. Cook for about 6 minutes per side, turning and brushing occasionally, until the chicken reaches an internal temperature of 165°F and the juices run clear.

5. Serve drizzled with the reserved sauce.

Technique tip: If using wooden skewers, prepare the skewers before using by soaking them in cold water for 1 hour to prevent scorching.

Per serving: *Calories: 252; Total Fat: 3g; Saturated Fat: 1g; Cholesterol: 80mg; Carbohydrates: 31g; Fiber: 1g; Protein: 26g*

Dairy-free, Nut-free

HAWAIIAN-INSPIRED HULI HULI CHICKEN

Serves 4 · **Prep time:** 10 minutes · **Cook time:** 20 minutes

Huli huli sauce originated in Hawaii, and it means "turned," which indicates the method of cooking the chicken: turning it and brushing with sauce as it cooks. It creates a sticky, coated chicken that's flavorful and delicious.

1 cup pineapple juice

¼ cup pure
maple syrup

¼ cup ketchup

2 tablespoons low-
sodium soy sauce
or tamari

1 teaspoon
ground ginger

1 teaspoon
garlic powder

4 bone-in, skin-on
chicken thighs

Olive oil, for greasing
the grill

1. In a medium bowl, whisk together the pine-apple juice, maple syrup, ketchup, soy sauce, ginger, and garlic powder.

2. Place the chicken in a resealable bag with the sauce. Marinate in the refrigerator for 1 hour. Remove the chicken from the sauce and pat dry. Pour the sauce into a saucepan.

3. Bring the sauce to a boil and simmer for about 10 minutes, stirring, until it is thick.

4. Heat a grill on medium-high and brush it with olive oil.

5. Place the chicken on the grill. Cook for about 30 minutes, turning occasionally and basting with the sauce, until it reaches an internal temperature of 165°F and the juices run clear.

Per serving: *Calories: 347; Total Fat: 19g; Saturated Fat: 5g; Cholesterol: 110mg; Carbohydrates: 26g; Fiber: <1g; Protein: 20g*

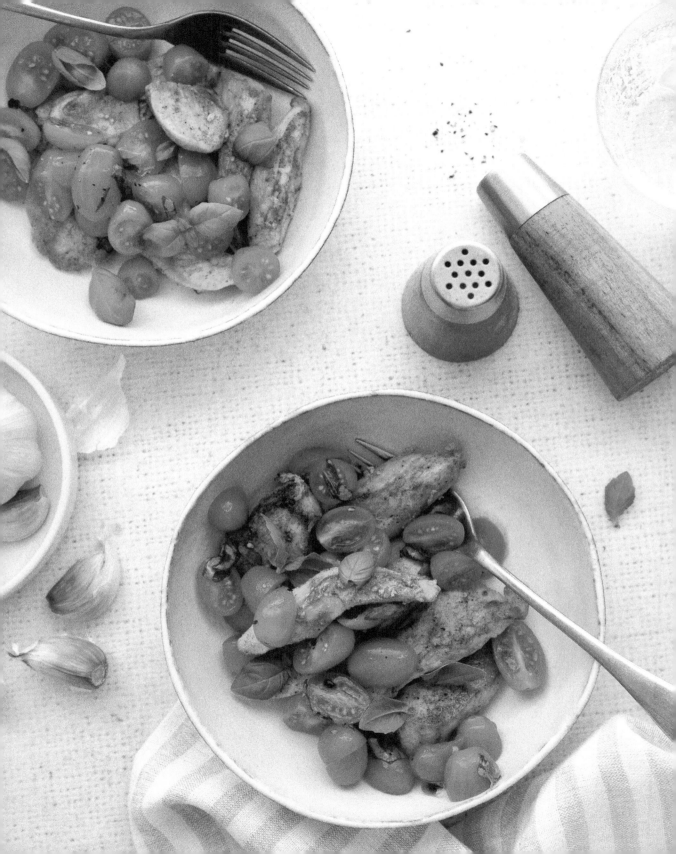

BRUSCHETTA CHICKEN BREAST

Serves 4 · **Prep time:** 10 minutes · **Cook time:** 20 minutes

You can prepare chicken breast quickly by cutting it into pieces and cooking it in a skillet in olive oil. Then serve it with the bruschetta topping for a delicious meal. If you make this ahead of time, store the chicken and bruschetta separately and reheat the chicken breast before serving.

1 pint cherry tomatoes, halved

¼ cup balsamic vinegar

3 tablespoons extra-virgin olive oil, divided

2 garlic cloves, minced

10 basil leaves, cut into strips

1 teaspoon sea salt, divided

1 pound boneless, skinless chicken breast, cut into 1-inch pieces

¼ teaspoon freshly ground black pepper

1. In a large bowl, combine the tomatoes, vinegar, 1 tablespoon of olive oil, the garlic, basil, and ½ teaspoon of salt. Mix well and set aside to allow the flavors to blend.

2. In a large skillet or sauté pan, heat the remaining 2 tablespoons of olive oil on medium-high until it shimmers.

3. Season the chicken with the remaining ½ teaspoon of salt and the pepper. Cook for 7 to 10 minutes, stirring occasionally, until cooked through.

4. Serve topped with the tomato mixture.

Variation tip: You can also toss the chicken with cooked whole-wheat pasta (2-ounce servings) and then toss that with the tomato mixture.

Per serving: *Calories: 249; Total Fat: 13g; Saturated Fat: 2g; Cholesterol: 80mg; Carbohydrates: 6g; Fiber: 1g; Protein: 26g*

Dairy-free, Nut-free

GROUND CHICKEN LETTUCE WRAPS

Serves 4 · **Prep time:** 10 minutes · **Cook time:** 15 minutes

Butter lettuce is the ideal lettuce to make wraps with because it has large, pliable, tender leaves. If you can't find butter lettuce, then romaine will do in a pinch, but the leaves aren't as pliable. You can make these ahead of time and reheat; store the chicken mixture separately from the lettuce and assemble when it's time to eat them.

2 tablespoons extra-virgin olive oil

1 pound ground chicken breast

8 ounces shiitake mushrooms, sliced

1 yellow onion, chopped

1 red bell pepper, sliced

¼ cup freshly squeezed orange juice

2 tablespoons low-sodium soy sauce

1 teaspoon ground ginger

1 teaspoon garlic powder

8 large butter lettuce leaves

1. In a large nonstick skillet or sauté pan, heat the olive oil on medium-high until it shimmers. Add the ground chicken and cook for about 6 minutes, crumbling with a spoon, until it is browned.

2. Using a slotted spoon, remove the chicken from the pan and set it aside on a platter. Add the mushrooms, onion, and pepper to the pan and cook for about 5 minutes, stirring occasionally, until the vegetables are soft. Return the chicken to the pan.

3. In a small bowl, whisk together the orange juice, soy sauce, ginger, and garlic powder. Add to the pan and bring to a simmer. Cook for about 3 minutes more, stirring, until the sauce is reduced.

4. Serve the chicken mixture wrapped in lettuce leaves.

Serving tip: Add garnishes if you wish, including 1 tablespoon of chopped almonds (per wrap) and thinly sliced scallions.

Per serving: *Calories: 286; Total Fat: 9g; Saturated Fat: 2g; Cholesterol: 80mg; Carbohydrates: 12g; Fiber: 3g; Protein: 28g*

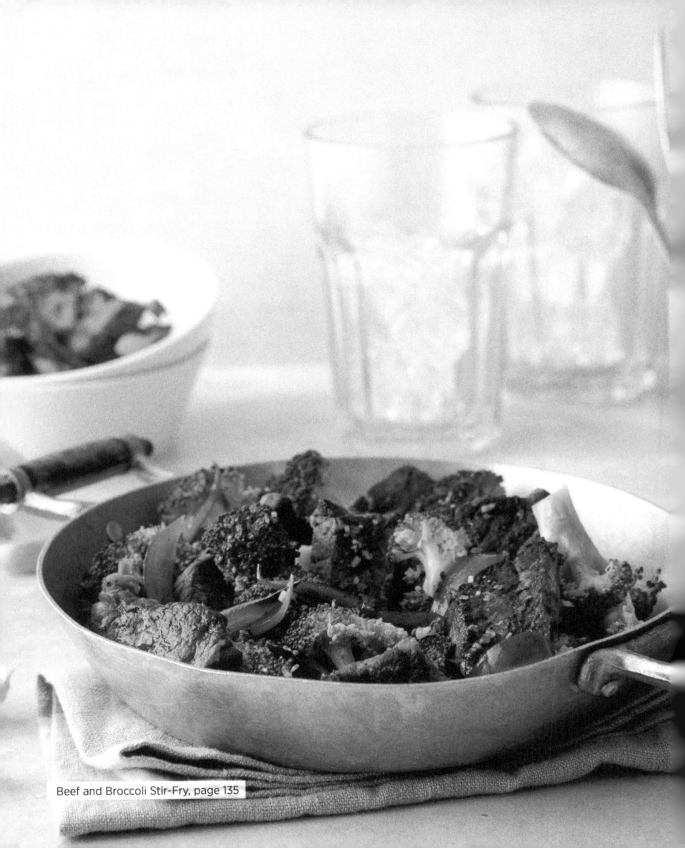

Beef and Broccoli Stir-Fry, page 135

Beef & Pork Mains

SPAGHETTI AND MEATBALLS

Serves 4 · **Prep time:** 15 minutes · **Cook time:** 20 minutes

Spaghetti and meatballs is a classic family favorite. The step in which you mix the milk and bread crumbs and allow them to soak together is called a *panade*, and it's essential to making moist meatballs, especially when you're working with extra-lean meats.

8 ounces whole-wheat spaghetti

½ cup unsweetened plain almond milk or skim milk

½ cup whole-wheat bread crumbs

12 ounces extra-lean ground beef

2 tablespoon dried Italian herbs, divided

2 teaspoons garlic powder, divided

1 teaspoon sea salt, divided

2 tablespoons extra-virgin olive oil

1 yellow onion, chopped

1 (28-ounce) can chopped tomatoes and basil, drained

1. Bring a large pot of water to a boil and cook the spaghetti according to the package directions. Drain and set aside.

2. Meanwhile, in a large bowl, combine the milk and bread crumbs. Mix well and allow the mixture to sit for 10 minutes for the milk and bread crumbs to combine.

3. Add the ground beef, 1 tablespoon of Italian herbs, 1 teaspoon of garlic powder, and ½ teaspoon of salt. Form into 1-inch meatballs.

4. In a large pot, heat the olive oil on medium-high until it shimmers. Add the meatballs and cook for about 8 minutes, turning occasionally, until the internal temperature reaches 160°F. Using a slotted spoon, remove the meatballs from the pot and set them aside on a platter.

5. Add the onion to the pot and cook for about 5 minutes, stirring occasionally, until soft.

6. In a blender or food processor, combine the tomatoes and the remaining 1 tablespoon of Italian herbs, 1 teaspoon of garlic powder, and ½ teaspoon of salt. Blend until smooth. Pour into the pan with the onions and bring to a simmer.

7. Return the meatballs to the pot. Bring to a simmer and reduce the heat to medium-low. Simmer for 5 minutes, stirring occasionally.

8. Spoon the sauce and meatballs over the hot noodles to serve.

Substitution tip: You can also make this gluten-free. Replace the bread crumbs with an equal amount of either gluten-free bread crumbs or almond flour, and replace the spaghetti with either zucchini noodles (cook them for about 5 minutes in the hot sauce), or with gluten-free spaghetti noodles.

Per serving: *Calories: 497; Total Fat: 13g; Saturated Fat: 3g; Cholesterol: 53mg; Carbohydrates: 69g; Fiber: 11g; Protein: 30g*

BEEF STREET-TACO SALAD

Serves 4 · **Prep time:** 15 minutes, plus 2 hours to marinate ·
Cook time: 20 minutes

Often, street tacos are topped with a slaw and put in soft corn tortillas. This salad ditches the corn tortillas and instead combines flank steak with a slightly spicy, creamy slaw.

6 scallions, both white and green parts, chopped, divided

¼ cup chopped fresh cilantro

Juice of 3 limes

4 tablespoons extra-virgin olive oil, divided

3 garlic cloves, chopped

1 teaspoon chipotle chili powder

¾ teaspoon sea salt, divided

1 (1-pound) flank steak

¼ cup nonfat plain Greek yogurt

1 (10-ounce) bag tri-color coleslaw mix

1. In a blender or food processor, combine 4 tablespoons of the scallions with the cilantro, lime juice, 2 tablespoons of olive oil, the garlic, chili powder, and ½ teaspoon of salt. Pulse for 20 (1-second) pulses. Set aside 2 tablespoons of the mixture and rub the rest all over the outside of the beef. Refrigerate the beef for 2 to 4 hours.

2. Mix the remaining 2 tablespoons of the herb mixture with the yogurt and refrigerate it.

3. After the meat has marinated, wipe off any excess marinade.

4. In a large nonstick skillet or sauté pan, heat the remaining 2 tablespoons of olive oil on medium-high until it shimmers. Add the meat and cook for about 7 minutes per side, turning once, until the internal temperature reaches 145°F. Remove from the pan and let rest, tented with foil, for about 10 minutes.

5. Meanwhile, in a large bowl, combine the slaw, the reserved scallions, and the herb–yogurt mixture. Toss to combine.

6. Cut the steak into thin slices, cutting against the grain. Serve the slaw with the meat on top.

Technique tip: Slicing the meat against the grain makes a tougher cut of meat tender. In bright light, look at the cooked meat and you'll notice there are striations running along the top. Cut perpendicular to these strands.

Per serving: *Calories: 352; Total Fat: 23g; Saturated Fat: 6g; Cholesterol: 54mg; Carbohydrates: 10g; Fiber: 3g; Protein: 28g*

Nut-free

MINI MEAT LOAVES WITH TOMATO GLAZE

Serves 4 · **Prep time:** 20 minutes · **Cook time:** 30 minutes

Meat loaf is a traditional family favorite. Serve this simple glazed meat loaf with a salad, slaw, or a side of steamed veggies for a tasty supper that will please your whole family.

½ cup whole-wheat
   bread crumbs

½ cup skim milk or
   unsweetened plain
   nondairy milk
   of choice

2 tablespoons
   extra-virgin olive oil

1 yellow onion, grated

½ cup ketchup

¼ cup apple cider
   vinegar

¼ cup pure
   maple syrup

½ teaspoon sriracha
   (optional)

1 pound extra-lean
   ground beef

1 large egg, beaten

1 teaspoon
   garlic powder

1 teaspoon dried thyme

1 teaspoon Dijon
   mustard

1 teaspoon sea salt

1. Preheat the oven to 350°F.

2. In a large bowl, combine the bread crumbs and milk. Mix well and let the mixture rest for 10 minutes.

3. In a large skillet or sauté pan, heat the olive oil on medium-high until it shimmers. Add the onion and cook for 5 minutes, stirring occasionally, until soft. Set aside to cool for 5 to 10 minutes.

4. In a small saucepan, whisk together the ketchup, vinegar, maple syrup, and sriracha (if using). Bring to a simmer for 5 minutes, stirring frequently, until thickened. Remove from the heat.

5. Add the cooled onions to the bowl with the bread crumbs and milk. Add the ground beef, egg, garlic powder, thyme, mustard, and salt. Mix well.

6. Divide the mixture into 8 portions and put in a 12-cup muffin tin; 4 of the tins will be empty (you can put water in them to prevent scorching). Brush the tops of the meat loaves with the glaze.

7. Bake for about 30 minutes, until the internal temperature reaches 160°F and the meat loaf is cooked through.

Technique tip: You can also cook this as a single meat loaf in a loaf pan. You'll need to increase the cooking time to about an hour.

Per serving (2 meat loaves): *Calories: 376; Total Fat: 13g; Saturated Fat: 3g; Cholesterol: 117mg; Carbohydrates: 36g; Fiber: 2g; Protein: 29g*

STEAK CHIMICHURRI

Serves 4 · **Prep time:** 10 minutes · **Cook time:** 15 minutes

Chimichurri is a sauce from Argentina that adds piquancy to meats, particularly steak. You can make the chimichurri ahead of time, store it in the refrigerator for up to 3 days, and then simply combine it with the cooked steak when you're ready to enjoy it.

½ cup chopped fresh Italian parsley

¼ cup chopped fresh cilantro

¼ cup chopped fresh oregano

¼ cup red wine vinegar

1 shallot, finely minced

4 tablespoons extra-virgin olive oil, divided

3 garlic cloves, minced

1 teaspoon sea salt, divided

¼ teaspoon red pepper flakes (optional)

1 (1-pound) flank steak

1. In a blender or food processor, combine the parsley, cilantro, oregano, vinegar, shallot, 2 tablespoons of olive oil, the garlic, ½ teaspoon of salt, and the red pepper flakes (if using). Pulse for 20 (1-second) pulses, until it resembles pesto. Refrigerate until ready to use.

2. Season the flank steak with the remaining ½ teaspoon of sea salt.

3. In a large nonstick skillet or sauté pan, heat the remaining 2 tablespoons of olive oil on medium-high until it shimmers. Add the steak and cook for about 7 minutes per side, until it reaches an internal temperature of 145°F. Let it rest for 10 minutes.

4. Slice the steak into thin strips against the grain. Serve with the chimichurri spooned over the top.

Substitution tip: Chimichurri is also good on grilled portobello mushrooms, if you'd prefer a vegetarian version of this dish.

Per serving: *Calories: 325; Total Fat: 23g; Saturated Fat: 6g; Cholesterol: 53mg; Carbohydrates: 4g; Fiber: 1g; Protein: 25g*

BEEF AND BROCCOLI STIR-FRY

Serves 4 · **Prep time:** 15 minutes · **Cook time:** 22 minutes

This Asian-inspired stir-fry is a classic combination of beef and broccoli. Serve it on cooked brown rice or cooked cauliflower rice for a full, satisfying meal.

2 tablespoons
   extra-virgin olive oil

1 pound sirloin steak,
   cut into 1-inch strips

2 cups broccoli florets

1 red onion,
   thinly sliced

1 tablespoon peeled
   and grated
   fresh ginger

3 garlic cloves, minced

2 tablespoons low-
   sodium soy sauce
   or tamari

Juice of 1 lime

½ teaspoon sesame oil

½ teaspoon red pepper
   flakes (optional)

1. In a large skillet or sauté pan, heat the olive oil on medium-high until it shimmers. Add the steak and cook for about 7 minutes, stirring occasionally, until it is browned. Using a slotted spoon, remove the steak from the oil and set it aside.

2. Add the broccoli, onion, and ginger to the oil in the pan. Cook for about 7 minutes, stirring, until the vegetables are crisp-tender. Add the garlic and cook, stirring constantly, for 30 seconds, until fragrant.

3. In a small bowl, whisk together the soy sauce, lime juice, sesame oil, and red pepper flakes (if using).

4. Return the beef to the pan and add the soy sauce mixture. Bring to a simmer. Cook for about 5 minutes more, stirring, until the liquid reduces.

Technique tip: To make cauliflower rice, split a head of cauliflower into florets and put them in a food processor. Pulse for 20 to 30 (1-second) pulses until it resembles rice. Alternatively, you can grate the cauliflower on a box grater. Cook in 2 tablespoons of olive oil for 5 to 7 minutes, until soft.

Per serving: *Calories: 256; Total Fat: 13g; Saturated Fat: 3g; Cholesterol: 58mg; Carbohydrates: 8g; Fiber: 2g; Protein: 29g*

GINGER-CILANTRO MEATBALLS

Serves 4 · **Prep time:** 15 minutes · **Cook time:** 30 minutes

These Asian-inspired meatballs make a delicious main course. Serve them with brown rice and steamed veggies or a simple side salad for a complete, nutritious, low-calorie meal.

1 pound extra-lean ground beef

1 cup shredded green cabbage

6 scallions, both white and green parts, finely chopped

½ cup chopped fresh cilantro

2 tablespoons peeled and grated fresh ginger

3 garlic cloves, minced

1 teaspoon fish sauce

½ teaspoon sriracha (optional)

1. Preheat the oven to 350°F. Line a rimmed baking sheet with parchment paper.

2. In a large bowl, combine the ground beef, cabbage, scallions, cilantro, ginger, garlic, fish sauce, and sriracha (if using). Mix well.

3. Form into 1-inch meatballs and place on the prepared baking sheet. Bake for about 30 minutes, until the internal temperature reaches 165°F and meat is no longer pink.

Technique tip: It's easiest to mix meatballs with very clean hands; it blends all the ingredients together much more thoroughly than trying to use a spoon.

Per serving: *Calories: 164; Total Fat: 5g; Saturated Fat: 2g; Cholesterol: 70mg; Carbohydrates: 5g; Fiber: 1g; Protein: 25g*

Nut-free

EASY PUB-STYLE BURGERS

Serves 4 · **Prep time:** 15 minutes · **Cook time:** 25 minutes

The secret to these burgers is the pub sauce and the caramelized onions, which turn a plain burger into a super flavorful one.

1 pound extra-lean ground beef

2 tablespoons pure maple syrup, divided

1 tablespoon low-sodium soy sauce, divided

1 teaspoon fish sauce, divided

1 teaspoon sea salt, divided

2 garlic cloves, minced, divided

2 tablespoons extra-virgin olive oil

2 yellow onions, thinly sliced

¼ cup nonfat plain Greek yogurt

4 whole-wheat hamburger buns, toasted

1. Preheat the oven to 425°F. Place a rack on a rimmed baking sheet.

2. In a large bowl, combine the ground beef, 1 tablespoon of maple syrup, ½ tablespoon of soy sauce, ½ teaspoon of fish sauce, ½ teaspoon of salt, and 1 garlic clove. Mix well and form into 4 patties. Place on the prepared baking sheet.

3. Bake the burgers for about 25 minutes, until they reach an internal temperature of 165°F and are cooked through.

4. Meanwhile, in a large skillet, heat the olive oil on medium-high until it shimmers. Add the onions and the remaining ½ teaspoon of salt and reduce the heat to low. Cook for about 20 minutes, stirring every 2 to 3 minutes, until the onions are browned and caramelized.

5. In a small bowl, whisk together the Greek yogurt, the remaining 1 tablespoon of maple syrup, ½ tablespoon of soy sauce, ½ teaspoon of fish sauce, and minced garlic clove. Mix well.

6. Serve the burgers on the buns, topped with the caramelized onions and the pub sauce.

Per serving: *Calories: 391; Total Fat: 13g; Saturated Fat: 3g; Cholesterol: 71mg; Carbohydrates: 38g; Fiber: 4g; Protein: 33g*

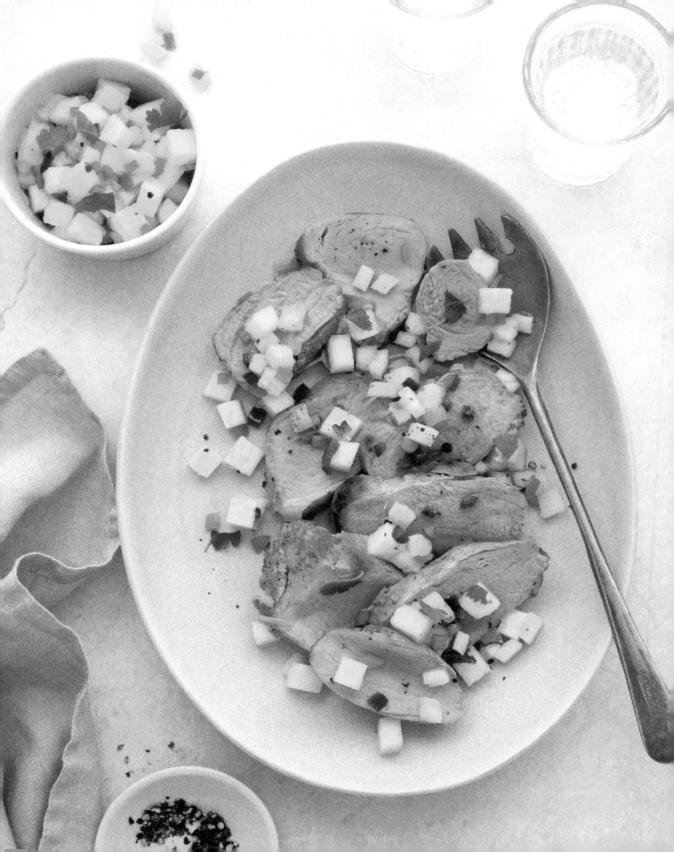

PORK TENDERLOIN WITH SPICY PINEAPPLE SAMBAL

Serves 4 · **Prep time:** 10 minutes · **Cook time:** 20 minutes

Pineapple sambal is inspired by the traditional Indonesian chili sauce. You can make it less spicy by using milder chiles than called for in the recipe, if you prefer. Prepare the sambal up to 3 days ahead of time and keep it in the refrigerator until you're ready to serve it.

1 (1-pound) pork tenderloin

¾ teaspoon sea salt, divided

¼ teaspoon freshly ground black pepper

2 tablespoons extra-virgin olive oil

1 shallot, minced

2 serrano or jalapeño peppers, seeds and ribs removed, minced

3 garlic cloves, minced

1 tablespoon fish sauce

2 cups chopped fresh pineapple

¼ cup chopped fresh cilantro

1. Preheat the oven to 400°F. Line a rimmed baking sheet with parchment paper.

2. Place the pork on the prepared baking sheet. Season with ½ teaspoon of salt and the black pepper. Roast for about 20 minutes, until it reaches an internal temperature of 145°F. Let rest for 10 minutes, tented with foil, before slicing.

3. Meanwhile, in a large skillet or sauté pan, heat the olive oil on medium-high until it shimmers. Add the shallot, serrano peppers, garlic, and remaining ¼ teaspoon of salt. Cook for about 7 minutes, stirring frequently, until the vegetables are very soft.

4. Add the fish sauce. Cook, stirring, for 3 minutes more. Let cool.

5. Stir in the pineapple and cilantro. Serve spooned over the sliced, cooked pork.

Substitution tip: While fresh pineapple tastes best here, to save time you can also purchase pre-chopped pineapple or canned pineapple packed in water and drained.

Per serving: *Calories: 238; Total Fat: 8g; Saturated Fat: 2g; Cholesterol: 64mg; Carbohydrates: 14g; Fiber: 2g; Protein: 26g*

Dairy-free, Gluten-free, Nut-free

MUSTARD AND HERB PORK TENDERLOIN

Serves 4 · **Prep time:** 10 minutes · **Cook time:** 20 minutes

Pork tenderloin is a lean cut of pork that, when cooked at a high temperature, remains juicy and delicious. Serve this with a simple fruit salad, fresh applesauce, coleslaw, or some grilled veggies of your choice for a delicious main dish.

¼ **cup fresh Italian parsley**

3 **tablespoons chopped fresh rosemary**

2 **tablespoons Dijon mustard**

2 **tablespoons apple cider vinegar**

2 **garlic cloves, minced**

½ **teaspoon sea salt**

¼ **teaspoon freshly ground black pepper**

1 **(1-pound) pork tenderloin**

1. Preheat the oven to 400°F. Line a rimmed baking sheet with parchment paper.

2. In a blender or food processor, combine the parsley, rosemary, mustard, vinegar, garlic, salt, and pepper. Pulse for 10 to 20 (1-second) pulses until it forms a paste. Spread on the outside of the pork tenderloin and place it on the prepared baking sheet.

3. Bake for about 20 minutes, until it reaches an internal temperature of 145°F. Rest for 10 minutes, tented with foil, before slicing and serving.

Technique tip: Don't skip resting the meat. If you slice meat too soon after it comes out of the oven, it loses juices and becomes dry. Tent with foil to keep the meat warm while it rests.

Per serving: *Calories: 136; Total Fat: 2g; Saturated Fat: 1g; Cholesterol: 64mg; Carbohydrates: 2g; Fiber: 1g; Protein: 26g*

ITALIAN SAUSAGE AND BROCCOLI RABE PITA PIZZAS

Serves 4 · **Prep time:** 15 minutes · **Cook time:** 10 minutes

Pitas make a delicious and quick pizza crust, so you can easily put together a pizza for a nutritious weeknight meal. If you can't find broccoli rabe, you can also use broccolini as a substitute.

4 whole-wheat pita rounds

1 (14.5-ounce) can oregano, garlic, and basil tomato sauce

12 ounces bulk Italian sausage

3 cups broccoli rabe, cut into pieces

1 shallot, finely minced

3 garlic cloves, minced

½ cup shredded Parmesan cheese

1. Preheat the oven to 425°F.

2. Place the pitas on a rimmed baking sheet and spread with the tomato sauce.

3. In a large skillet or sauté pan, cook the Italian sausage for about 6 minutes, crumbling it with a spoon, until browned.

4. Add the broccoli rabe and shallot and cook for 3 to 4 minutes, stirring, until it is soft. Add the garlic and cook, stirring constantly, for 30 seconds, until fragrant.

5. Divide evenly among the pitas. Sprinkle with the cheese.

6. Bake for about 10 minutes, until the cheese is melted and beginning to brown.

Substitution tip: You can make these dairy-free by omitting the Parmesan cheese or using a vegan cheese in place of the Parmesan.

Per serving: *Calories: 523; Total Fat: 27g; Saturated Fat: 10g; Cholesterol: 79mg; Carbohydrates: 44g; Fiber: 8g; Protein: 29g*

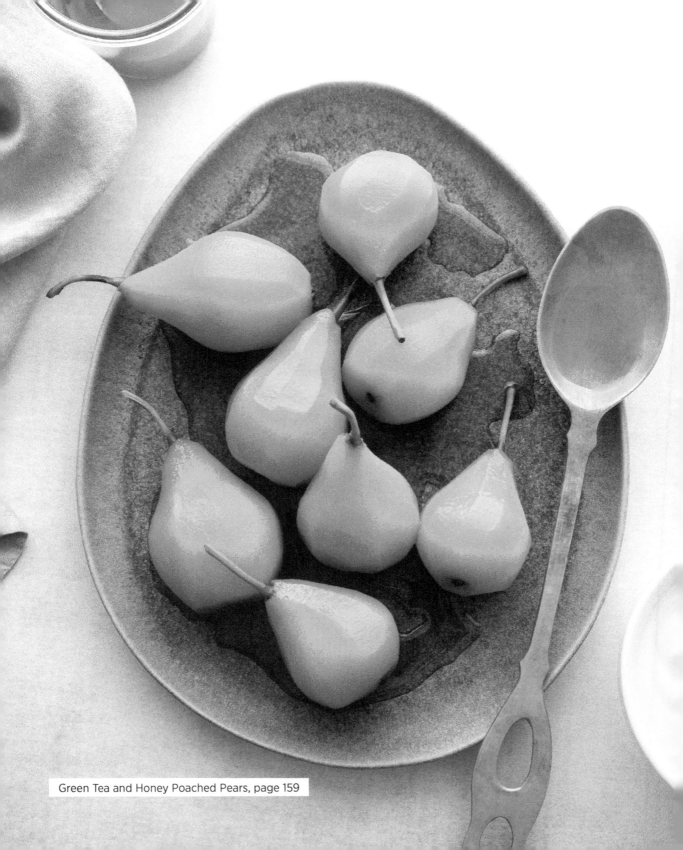

Green Tea and Honey Poached Pears, page 159

Snacks, Sides & Sweets

Dairy-free, Gluten-free, Nut-free, Vegan

CITRUS SPINACH

Serves 4 · **Prep time:** 10 minutes · **Cook time:** 10 minutes

Citrus adds bright flavors to this simple side dish. Baby spinach is packed with nutrients including folic acid and iron, and citrus juice adds vitamin C that helps your body better absorb the iron. Baby spinach is also more tender than fully grown spinach, which makes it ideal for a quick sauté.

2 tablespoons
extra-virgin olive oil

2 tablespoons minced
shallot

6 cups fresh
baby spinach

½ teaspoon sea salt

⅛ teaspoon freshly
ground black pepper

2 garlic cloves, minced

Juice of 1 orange

1. In a large skillet or sauté pan, heat the olive oil on medium-high until it shimmers. Add the shallot and cook for about 3 minutes, stirring, until the shallot is soft.

2. Add the spinach, salt, and pepper. Cook for about 2 minutes, stirring, until the spinach is wilted.

3. Add the garlic and cook, stirring constantly, for 30 seconds, until fragrant.

4. Add the orange juice and cook for about 5 minutes more, stirring occasionally, until the juice is reduced and syrupy.

Substitution tip: Change the flavor profile by replacing the orange juice with ¼ cup of balsamic or red wine vinegar and 1 tablespoon of honey.

Per serving: *Calories: 86; Total Fat: 7g; Saturated Fat: 1g; Cholesterol: 0mg; Carbohydrates: 5g; Fiber: 1g; Protein: 2g*

Dairy-free, Gluten-free, Nut-free, Vegetarian

ROASTED BALSAMIC BRUSSELS SPROUTS

Serves 4 · **Prep time:** 10 minutes · **Cook time:** 40 minutes

When you roast Brussels sprouts at a high temperature, they develop deep, warm, caramelized flavors that make a satisfying and flavorful side dish that's delicious with poultry or beef.

1½ pounds Brussels sprouts, halved

2 tablespoons extra-virgin olive oil

½ teaspoon sea salt

⅛ teaspoon freshly ground black pepper

½ cup balsamic vinegar

1 tablespoon honey

1. Preheat the oven to 400°F.

2. In a large bowl, toss the Brussels sprouts with the olive oil, salt, and pepper. Spread, cut-side down, on a large rimmed baking sheet in a single layer.

3. Roast for about 40 minutes, until the Brussels sprouts are browned and caramelized.

4. Meanwhile, in a small saucepan, combine the vinegar and honey. Bring to a simmer on medium-high and then reduce the heat to low. Simmer for 7 to 10 minutes, stirring occasionally, until the liquid is thick and syrupy. Drizzle over the cooked Brussels sprouts.

Technique tip: To prepare the Brussels sprouts, trim the ends, and halve the Brussels sprouts. Rinse in a bowl of cold water and pat dry completely.

Per serving: *Calories: 177; Total Fat: 7g; Saturated Fat: 1g; Cholesterol: 0mg; Carbohydrates: 25g; Fiber: 7g; Protein: 6g*

Dairy-free, Gluten-free, Vegan

GREEN BEANS AND RED BELL PEPPERS

Serves 4 · **Prep time:** 10 minutes · **Cook time:** 12 minutes

Blanching the green beans before sautéing helps keep them brightly colored and tender. Once the beans are blanched, this is a quick and colorful stir-fry that's a perfect veggie side, and with its bright red and green color, it's an effective stir-fry for the holidays.

1 pound fresh green beans, cut into 1-inch pieces

2 tablespoons extra-virgin olive oil

2 tablespoons minced shallot

1 red bell pepper, chopped

½ teaspoon sea salt

⅛ teaspoon freshly ground black pepper

Juice and zest of ½ lemon

2 tablespoons pine nuts (optional)

1. Bring a large pot of water to a boil and prepare a large bowl with ice water. Once the water is boiling, cook the beans for 2 minutes in the water. Plunge the beans into the ice water bath to stop the cooking. Drain.

2. In a large skillet or sauté pan, heat the olive oil on medium-high until it shimmers. Add the shallot and cook for 2 minutes, stirring, until softened.

3. Add the beans, bell pepper, salt, and black pepper. Cook for about 5 minutes, stirring, until the vegetables are tender.

4. Add the lemon juice and zest and pine nuts (if using). Cook, stirring, for 2 minutes more.

Variation tip: This dish is delicious with a light cheesy flavor. Garnish with up to 2 tablespoons of shredded Parmesan cheese or nutritional yeast.

Per serving: *Calories: 109; Total Fat: 7g; Saturated Fat: 1g; Cholesterol: 0mg; Carbohydrates: 11g; Fiber: 4g; Protein: 3g*

Dairy-free, Gluten-free, Nut-free, Vegan

CAULIFLOWER RICE

Serves 4 · **Prep time:** 10 minutes · **Cook time:** 5 minutes

Cauliflower rice makes a tasty side dish, and it is a good low-calorie and low-carb alternative to brown rice. You can make it in large batches and freeze it for up to 6 months in 1-cup servings.

1 head cauliflower, cut into florets

2 tablespoons extra-virgin olive oil

½ teaspoon sea salt

1. In a blender or food processor, pulse the cauliflower florets with 1-second pulses until they resemble rice. Alternatively, grate the cauliflower on a box grater.

2. In a large skillet or sauté pan, heat the olive oil on medium-high until it shimmers.

3. Add the cauliflower and salt and cook for about 5 minutes, or until the cauliflower is tender.

Substitution tip: Add some color and flavor to this rice with broccoli. Replace up to half the cauliflower with broccoli florets.

Per serving: *Calories: 96; Total Fat: 7g; Saturated Fat: 1g; Cholesterol: 0mg; Carbohydrates: 7g; Fiber: 3g; Protein: 3g*

SOUTHWESTERN SALSA FRESCA

Serves 4 · **Prep time:** 10 minutes

You can use this simple fresh salsa as a dip for baked corn tortillas, on top of fish or poultry, or to spice up cauliflower or brown rice for a colorful and tasty side dish. Use the freshest ingredients possible to make this a truly flavorful sauce.

1 pint cherry tomatoes, finely chopped

½ red onion, finely chopped

¼ cup chopped fresh cilantro

Juice of ½ lime

1 jalapeño pepper, ribs and seeds removed, minced

1 garlic clove, minced

½ teaspoon sea salt

In a medium bowl, combine the tomatoes, onion, cilantro, lime juice, jalapeño, garlic, and salt. Let sit at room temperature for about 20 minutes before serving to allow the flavors to blend.

Substitution tip: You can replace the tomatoes with 2 cups of chopped fruit, such as mango, papaya, or melon, to make a delicious fruit salsa.

Per serving: *Calories: 22; Total Fat: <1g; Saturated Fat: 0g; Cholesterol: 0mg; Carbohydrates: 5g; Fiber: 1g; Protein: 1g*

Dairy-free, Gluten-free, Nut-free, Vegan

HUMMUS AND RED BELL PEPPER STICKS

Serves 4 · **Prep time:** 10 minutes

Hummus makes a delicious snack. This Middle Eastern chickpea spread is flavorful and delicious as a spread for vegetables, sandwiches, and more. You should be able to find tahini near the peanut butter at the grocery store.

1 (15-ounce) can chickpeas, drained and rinsed

Juice of 1 lemon

2 tablespoons extra-virgin olive oil

1 tablespoon tahini

2 garlic cloves, minced

½ teaspoon sea salt

2 red bell peppers, cut into strips

1. In a blender or food processor, combine the chickpeas, lemon juice, olive oil, tahini, garlic, and salt. Blend until smooth.

2. Serve with the bell peppers for dipping.

Variation tip: Make a tasty red pepper hummus by adding 2 to 3 pieces of jarred roasted red pepper to the hummus in step 1.

Per serving: *Calories: 195; Total Fat: 11g; Saturated Fat: 1g; Cholesterol: 0mg; Carbohydrates: 21g; Fiber: 6g; Protein: 6g*

Dairy-free, Gluten-free, Nut-free, Vegan

GUACAMOLE AND JICAMA

Serves 4 · **Prep time:** 10 minutes

Guacamole is a fast and easy mashed avocado sauce that's great with southwestern-flavored foods, as well as being a delicious dip for jicama or other sliced crisp veggies. Choose avocados that yield to pressure when gently pressed without being super mushy.

1 avocado, pitted, peeled, and chopped

¼ red onion, minced

2 tablespoons chopped fresh cilantro

Juice of 1 lime

1 garlic clove, minced

¼ teaspoon sea salt

1 jicama, peeled and cut into sticks

1. In a small bowl, combine the avocado, onion, cilantro, lime juice, garlic, and salt. Mash with a fork.

2. Serve right away with the jicama for dipping.

Technique tip: Use a vegetable peeler to peel the jicama. Trim the jicama with a sharp knife to remove the rounded edges (you can chop and add them to a salad) and cut the vegetable into a cube. Then cut lengthwise and crosswise into sticks.

Per serving: *Calories: 126; Total Fat: 5g; Saturated Fat: 1g; Cholesterol: 0mg; Carbohydrates: 19g; Fiber: 11g; Protein: 2g*

SPICED ROASTED CHICKPEAS

Serves 4 · **Prep time:** 5 minutes · **Cook time:** 20 minutes

Chickpeas have a starchy texture that make them satisfyingly crispy when roasted. These snacks will keep for up to 1 week when stored tightly sealed at room temperature, so they're perfect snacks for on the go.

1 (15-ounce) can chickpeas, drained, rinsed, and patted dry

2 tablespoons extra-virgin olive oil

½ teaspoon garlic powder

½ teaspoon ground cumin

½ teaspoon smoked paprika

½ teaspoon sea salt

¼ teaspoon ground cinnamon

1. Preheat the oven to 400°F. Line a rimmed baking sheet with parchment paper.

2. In a large bowl, combine the chickpeas, olive oil, garlic powder, cumin, paprika, salt, and cinnamon. Toss to mix.

3. Spread in an even layer on the baking sheet and cook for about 20 minutes, stirring occasionally, until the chickpeas are crisp.

Technique tip: Drying the chickpeas as much as possible is essential for crispy chickpeas. Drain and rinse them in a colander and allow them to sit for about 30 minutes. Then put them on a paper towel or tea towel and pat them dry.

Per serving: *Calories: 157; Total Fat: 9g; Saturated Fat: 1g; Cholesterol: 0mg; Carbohydrates: 16g; Fiber: 4g; Protein: 5g*

Dairy-free, Gluten-free, Nut-free, Vegan

BAKED SWEET POTATO CHIPS

Serves 4 · **Prep time:** 10 minutes · **Cook time:** 30 minutes

The trick to crispy baked chips is super thinly sliced potatoes. If you have a mandoline or a slicer attachment to a food processor, this can ensure that the chips are super thin. Otherwise, use a sharp knife and a steady hand to make the thinnest slices you can manage.

2 sweet potatoes, very thinly sliced

2 tablespoons extra-virgin olive oil

½ teaspoon sea salt

1. Preheat the oven to 300°F. Line two large rimmed baking sheets with parchment paper.

2. In a large bowl, combine the sweet potatoes, olive oil, and salt. Toss to mix.

3. Spread in an even layer on the prepared baking sheets and bake for about 30 minutes, until crisp. Let cool before serving.

Technique tip: If you don't have a mandoline or slicer attachment, you can also use a vegetable peeler to create thin slices. The thinner the slices, the crispier the chips.

Per serving: *Calories: 116; Total Fat: 7g; Saturated Fat: 1g; Cholesterol: 0mg; Carbohydrates: 13g; Fiber: 2g; Protein: 1g*

Dairy-free, Gluten-free, Nut-free, Vegan

SESAME-GINGER KALE CHIPS

Serves 4 · **Prep time:** 10 minutes · **Cook time:** 55 minutes

Kale chips are light and crispy, and the sesame adds a nice toasted flavor to them. They're also a nutritious alternative to commercial chips. These will store, tightly sealed, for up to 5 days.

1 bunch fresh kale, stemmed and torn into 2-inch pieces

¼ cup sesame seeds

2 tablespoons extra-virgin olive oil

1 tablespoon peeled and grated fresh ginger

½ teaspoon sesame oil

½ teaspoon sea salt

1. Preheat the oven to 200°F. Line two large rimmed baking sheets with parchment paper.

2. In a large bowl, combine the kale, sesame seeds, olive oil, ginger, sesame oil, and salt. Toss to mix.

3. Spread in an even layer on the prepared baking sheets and bake for 30 minutes. Flip and cook for about 25 minutes more on the other side until crisp.

Technique tip: You can also use this recipe to make chips from Swiss chard or collard greens, which have a similar texture to but slightly different flavors from kale.

Per serving: *Calories: 139; Total Fat: 14g; Saturated Fat: 2g; Cholesterol: 0mg; Carbohydrates: 3g; Fiber: 3g; Protein: 3g*

EASY REFRIGERATOR DILL PICKLES

Serves 4 · **Prep time:** 10 minutes · **Cook time:** 5 minutes

When cucumbers are in season, there's nothing better than a homemade dill pickle. These simple refrigerator dill pickles skip the canning process, so they're quick and easy. You'll need to refrigerate them for about 1 week before they're ready to eat. They'll keep in the refrigerator, sealed, for up to 1 month.

4 cups
   cucumber spears

1 cup roughly chopped
   fresh dill

4 garlic cloves, minced

3 cups water

1¾ cups red wine
   vinegar

1 tablespoon sea salt

1. In jars, a large crock, or a bowl you can cover, combine the cucumbers, dill, and garlic.

2. In a large saucepan, combine the water, vinegar, and salt. Bring to a boil and then remove from the heat and cool completely.

3. Pour the liquid over the cucumbers. Seal and refrigerate for 1 week.

Variation tip: Prefer a more garlicky pickle? Like a spicy pickle? Add as much garlic as you like—the 4 cloves are just a suggestion. To make a spicier pickle, add red pepper flakes (up to ½ teaspoon or more if you like a lot of heat) to the vinegar mixture as it cooks.

Per serving: *Calories: 41; Total Fat: <1g; Saturated Fat: 0g; Cholesterol: 0mg; Carbohydrates: 5g; Fiber: 1g; Protein: 1g*

Gluten-free, Nut-free, Vegetarian

ROASTED RED PEPPER DEVILED EGGS

Serves 4 · **Prep time:** 10 minutes

Deviled eggs make a delicious appetizer or snack, and they even make a tasty breakfast or lunch. This version adds chopped roasted red peppers (you can buy them in a jar) to add color and flavor to a classic recipe.

8 hard-boiled eggs, cooled and peeled

¼ cup nonfat plain Greek yogurt

1 tablespoon mayonnaise

1 teaspoon Dijon mustard

1 teaspoon red wine vinegar

½ teaspoon sea salt

⅛ teaspoon freshly ground black pepper

¼ cup chopped jarred roasted red peppers

Smoked paprika, for garnish

1. Halve the eggs lengthwise and scoop out the yolks with a spoon. Place the whites on a plate, cut-side up, and place the yolks in a bowl.

2. Add to the yolks the yogurt, mayonnaise, mustard, vinegar, salt, and black pepper. Use a fork to smash and mix until well combined. Fold in the red peppers.

3. Spoon the yolk mixture into the whites and sprinkle with the paprika. These will keep for up to 3 days in the refrigerator.

Variation tip: Add 2 tablespoons of chopped, fresh tarragon to the yolks when you fold in the red peppers to add a lovely, herbal flavor.

Per serving: *Calories: 173; Total Fat: 12g; Saturated Fat: 3g; Cholesterol: 330mg; Carbohydrates: 2g; Fiber: 0g; Protein: 13g*

Dairy-free, Gluten-free, Vegan

CINNAMON BAKED APPLES

Serves 4 · **Prep time:** 10 minutes · **Cook time:** 50 minutes

Baked apples make a delicious dessert or side dish, especially with pork. These spiced apples would be a tasty, lighter stand-in for apple pie. Serve them warm.

4 apples, tops cut off and cores removed with the bottom left intact

¼ cup chopped pecans

3 tablespoons pure maple syrup

1 teaspoon ground cinnamon

1. Preheat the oven to 375°F.

2. Place the apples, cut-side up, in a baking pan.

3. In a medium bowl, combine the pecans, syrup, and cinnamon. Mix well. Spoon the mixture into the apples' cavities and bake for 40 to 45 minutes, or until soft.

Technique tip: Use a sharp paring knife to cut out the apple core without cutting through the bottom. Insert the knife along the edge of the core after you've cut the apple top off, and then cut around the core without piercing the bottom. Use a teaspoon to scoop out the core and round out the hole you've made in the apple.

Per serving: *Calories: 182; Total Fat: 5g; Saturated Fat: 1g; Cholesterol: 0mg; Carbohydrates: 37g; Fiber: 5g; Protein: 1g*

ALMOND BUTTER APPLE SANDWICHES

Serves 4 · **Prep time:** 10 minutes

Quick and easy, these simple apple sandwiches make tasty snacks, a yummy breakfast, or a delicious dessert. They're low in sugar but still lightly sweet and crispy—all the elements necessary for a simple and satisfying snack.

4 tablespoons almond butter

1 tablespoon pure maple syrup

2 apples, cored with top and bottom cut off and cut into 8 thick crosswise slices

1. In a small bowl, mix the almond butter and maple syrup until well blended.

2. Spread the mixture on 4 apple slices and top with the remaining 4 apple slices.

Variation tip: Add some salt to your sweet by sprinkling the almond butter with a large-grain salt after it has been spread on the apples. A little goes a long way—each will require just a pinch.

Per serving: *Calories: 156; Total Fat: 9g; Saturated Fat: 1g; Cholesterol: 0mg; Carbohydrates: 19g; Fiber: 4g; Protein: 4g*

Dairy-free, Vegan

NUT BUTTER ENERGY BALLS

Serves 4 · **Prep time:** 10 minutes

These nutritious and slightly sweet balls make a great snack, and they'll keep for up to 6 months in the freezer. They're sweetened with dates (you can find them in the produce section at the grocery store), so they are sweet without containing any refined sugar.

1 cup pitted
  Medjool dates

½ cup almond butter

½ cup old-
  fashioned oats

¼ cup pepitas

1 tablespoon
  chia seeds

2 teaspoons peeled
  and grated
  fresh ginger

Pinch salt

1. In a blender or food processor, combine the dates, almond butter, oats, pepitas, chia seeds, ginger, and salt. Pulse with 1-second pulses until well combined.

2. Roll into 1-inch balls and refrigerate or freeze until you're ready to serve. Store in the refrigerator for up to 5 days or in the freezer for up to 6 months.

Substitution tip: You can also use cashew butter or peanut butter (an equal amount) to make these balls. Make sure you purchase a natural, sugar-free nut butter. If you're allergic to nuts, you can use a seed butter such as SunButter.

Per serving: *Calories: 472; Total Fat: 23g; Saturated Fat: 2g; Cholesterol: 0mg; Carbohydrates: 65g; Fiber: 10g; Protein: 12g*

Dairy-free, Gluten-free, Nut-free, Vegetarian

GREEN TEA AND HONEY POACHED PEARS

Serves 4 · **Prep time:** 10 minutes · **Cook time:** 40 minutes

Pears have a lovely, delicate flavor that soaks up the sweetness of the honey and the slightly floral taste of green tea. Serve these warm as a dessert or use them to top plain, nonfat yogurt for a sweet treat.

2 cups brewed green tea

2 cups apple or pear juice

¼ cup honey

2 (1-inch) slices fresh ginger

½ teaspoon ground cinnamon

4 small pears, peeled

1. In a large pot, combine the tea, juice, honey, ginger, and cinnamon. Bring to a simmer on medium high.

2. Add the pears and simmer for 20 to 30 minutes, until tender. Remove the pears from the liquid and cool in the refrigerator.

3. Return the liquid to the heat and simmer for about 20 minutes more, stirring occasionally, until it is thick and syrupy. Cool and serve spooned over the pears.

Substitution tip: Use jasmine green tea for a lightly floral flavor.

Per serving: *Calories: 206; Total Fat:<1 g; Saturated Fat: 0g; Cholesterol: 0mg; Carbohydrates: 54g; Fiber: 5g; Protein: 1g*

Gluten-free, Nut-free, Vegetarian

HONEYED GREEK YOGURT WITH GINGER BERRY COMPOTE

Serves 4 · **Prep time:** 10 minutes · **Cook time:** 10 minutes

This is a simple yet flavorful dessert that's not too sweet. Store the cooked and cooled berries separately from the yogurt in the refrigerator for up to 1 week. You can also use frozen berries in place of fresh—just make sure they don't have sugar added.

1 pint blueberries

1 pint blackberries

Juice of 1 orange

2 tablespoons peeled and grated fresh ginger

1 cup plain nonfat or low-fat Greek yogurt

2 tablespoons honey

1. In a large saucepan, combine the berries, orange juice, and ginger. Bring to a simmer on medium-high and cook for about 10 minutes, stirring occasionally, until the fruit is soft and the liquid reduced. Cool completely.

2. Whisk together the yogurt and honey until well combined. Spoon into 4 bowls and top with the cooled berry compote.

Substitution tip: Make this vegan and dairy-free by substituting a plain, nondairy yogurt such as soy yogurt or almond milk yogurt.

Per serving: Calories: 159; Total Fat: 1g; Saturated Fat: <1g; Cholesterol: 3mg; Carbohydrates: 33g; Fiber: 6g; Protein: 8g

Dairy-free, Gluten-free, Vegetarian

ALMOND BUTTER CHOCOLATE CHIP COOKIES

Makes 10 cookies · **Prep time:** 10 minutes · **Cook time:** 10 minutes

These cookies have only a few ingredients, and because they don't contain flour, they're also naturally gluten-free. You'll find coconut sugar, which is a less refined version of sugar, in the baking section of your grocery store. Alternatively, you can use an erythritol-based granulated sugar substitute, such as Swerve, or a monk fruit granulated sweetener.

1 cup almond butter

¾ cup coconut sugar or granulated sugar substitute

1 large egg, beaten

½ cup dark chocolate chips

1. Preheat the oven to 350°F. Line a rimmed baking sheet with parchment paper and set aside.

2. In a large bowl, beat the almond butter, coconut sugar, and egg until well blended. Fold in the chocolate chips.

3. Form into 12 (1-inch) balls and place on a baking sheet. Flatten slightly. Bake for about 20 minutes, until golden brown.

4. Cool on the pan before lifting them off with a spatula. Store in an airtight container for up to 1 week at room temperature or freeze for up to 6 months.

Substitution tip: If you can find them, use a stevia-sweetened chocolate chip, such as those from Lily's, to make these even lower in sugar.

Per serving (1 cookie): *Calories: 225; Total Fat: 15g; Saturated Fat: 3g; Cholesterol: 16mg; Carbohydrates: 19g; Fiber: 3g; Protein: 6g*

Dairy-free, Gluten-free, Vegan

MAPLE-GINGER APPLESAUCE

Makes about 2 cups · **Prep time:** 10 minutes · **Cook time:** 20 minutes

Applesauce is a delicious dessert, whether you eat it plain or mix it with nonfat plain Greek yogurt. Use a combination of sweet-tart apples, such as two Granny Smith and two Braeburn apples. Avoid using Red Delicious apples or Golden Delicious apples, which are a bit too sweet for this applesauce.

4 apples, peeled, cored, and cut into chunks

½ cup water

¼ cup pure maple syrup

1 teaspoon ground cinnamon

1 teaspoon ground ginger

1. In a large pot, combine the apples, water, maple syrup, cinnamon, and ginger.

2. Bring to a simmer on medium-high, then reduce the heat to medium-low. Cover and simmer for 20 minutes, or until the apples are soft. Cool before serving.

3. Store in an airtight container for up to 5 days in the refrigerator or up to 6 months in the freezer.

Variation tip: Add ½ cup of fresh cranberries for a delicious apple cranberry sauce.

Per serving (½ cup): *Calories: 149; Total Fat: <1g; Saturated Fat: <1g; Cholesterol: 0mg; Carbohydrates: 39g; Fiber: 5g; Protein: 1g*

CREAMY MIXED BERRY FREEZER POPS

Makes 4 pops · **Prep time:** 5 minutes

These creamy freezer pops are simple and satisfying. You can use frozen mixed berries that you've thawed, or you can use fresh berries; either way, you'll need 4 cups total. If you're using frozen berries, make sure that they don't have added sugar.

4 cups mixed berries (strawberries, blueberries, blackberries, raspberries)

½ cup nonfat plain Greek yogurt

½ cup unsweetened plain almond milk or nondairy milk of choice

¼ cup honey

1. In a blender or food processor, combine the berries, yogurt, almond milk, and honey. Blend until smooth.

2. Pour into ice pop molds and freeze for at least 6 hours or up to 6 months.

Technique tip: Don't have ice pop molds? No problem! Pour into paper cups. Cover with aluminum foil and insert ice pop sticks through the foil. Freeze as indicated and peel away the paper cups when you serve.

Per serving (1 pop): *Calories: 154; Total Fat: 1g; Saturated Fat: <1g; Cholesterol: 2mg; Carbohydrates: 36g; Fiber: 3g; Protein: 4g*

Dairy-free, Gluten-free, Vegan

MAPLE-PECAN BAKED PEACHES

Serves 4 · **Prep time:** 5 minutes · **Cook time:** 30 minutes

Whether you serve them warm or cooled, these sweet spiced peaches make a delicious and satisfying dessert. They are also wonderful with ¼ cup of plain Greek yogurt that has 1 or 2 tablespoons of pure maple syrup whisked in.

4 peaches, halved and pitted

¼ cup pure maple syrup

¼ cup chopped pecans

½ teaspoon ground cinnamon

1. Preheat the oven to 350°F.

2. In a baking pan, place the peaches, cut-side up. Drizzle with the syrup and sprinkle with the pecans and cinnamon.

3. Bake for about 30 minutes, until the peaches are soft.

Substitution tip: Cardamom is also delicious on these peaches, although a little goes a long way. Mix about ¼ teaspoon of ground cardamom with the cinnamon before sprinkling it on the peaches.

Per serving: *Calories: 158; Total Fat: 5g; Saturated Fat: 1g; Cholesterol: 0mg; Carbohydrates: 29g; Fiber: 3g; Protein: 2g*

Dairy-free, Gluten-free, Vegetarian

BANANA ALMOND BUTTER "ICE CREAM"

Serves 4 · **Prep time:** 5 minutes

Bananas are a super-versatile ingredient, and they make a creamy non-dairy frozen dessert with a texture similar to ice cream. You'll need very ripe bananas; the browner the better, because that gives the sugars time to develop and makes the bananas both easy to mash and creamier.

4 very ripe bananas, peeled

2 tablespoons almond butter

1 tablespoon honey

½ teaspoon ground cinnamon

1. In a medium bowl, mash the bananas, almond butter, honey, and cinnamon and mix until well blended.

2. Freeze for 6 hours in an airtight container.

3. Transfer to a blender or food processor. Pulse for 1-second pulses until it is smooth and creamy; this will take about 5 minutes of pulsing, pausing to scrape down the sides of the container occasionally.

4. Freeze in an airtight container until solid, about 6 hours more. Store in the freezer for up to 6 months.

Variation tip: Add 1 tablespoon of unsweetened cocoa powder to make a chocolate banana ice cream.

Per serving: *Calories: 170; Total Fat: 5g; Saturated Fat: 1g; Cholesterol: 0mg; Carbohydrates: 33g; Fiber: 4g; Protein: 3g*

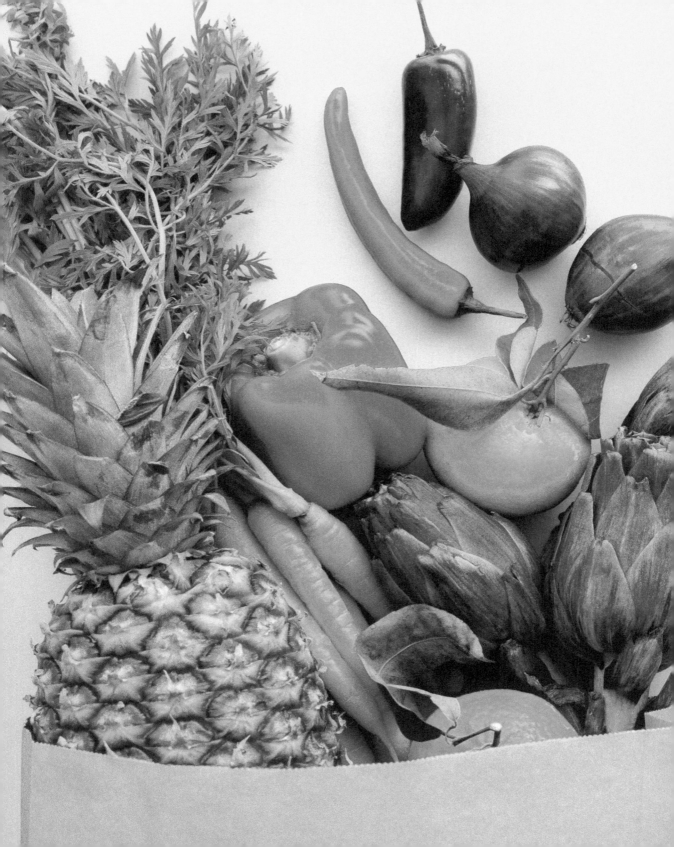

MEASUREMENT CONVERSIONS

OVEN TEMPERATURES

FAHRENHEIT	CELSIUS (APPROXIMATE)
250°F	120°C
300°F	150°C
325°F	165°C
350°F	180°C
375°F	190°C
400°F	200°C
425°F	220°C
450°F	230°C

VOLUME EQUIVALENTS (LIQUID)

US STANDARD	US STANDARD (OUNCES)	METRIC (APPROXIMATE)
2 tablespoons	1 fl. oz.	30 mL
¼ cup	2 fl. oz.	60 mL
½ cup	4 fl. oz.	120 mL
1 cup	8 fl. oz.	240 mL
1½ cups	12 fl. oz.	355 mL
2 cups or 1 pint	16 fl. oz.	475 mL
4 cups or 1 quart	32 fl. oz.	1 L
1 gallon	128 fl. oz.	4 L

WEIGHT EQUIVALENTS

US STANDARD	METRIC (APPROXIMATE)
½ ounce	15 g
1 ounce	30 g
2 ounces	60 g
4 ounces	115 g
8 ounces	225 g
12 ounces	340 g
16 ounces or 1 pound	455 g

VOLUME EQUIVALENTS (DRY)

US STANDARD	METRIC (APPROXIMATE)
⅛ teaspoon	0.5 mL
¼ teaspoon	1 mL
½ teaspoon	2 mL
¾ teaspoon	4 mL
1 teaspoon	5 mL
1 tablespoon	15 mL
¼ cup	59 mL
⅓ cup	79 mL
½ cup	118 mL
⅔ cup	156 mL
¾ cup	177 mL
1 cup	235 mL
2 cups or 1 pint	475 mL
3 cups	700 mL
4 cups or 1 quart	1 L

RESOURCES

For general information regarding nutrition, refer to the United States Department of Agriculture's (USDA) Choose MyPlate (MyPlate. gov) as well as the Dietary Guidelines (DietaryGuidelines.gov).

For more information regarding physical activity guidelines for Americans, visit the US Department of Health and Human Services website Health.gov/our-work/physical-activity/current-guidelines.

REFERENCES

Clark, Michael, Brian G. Sutton, and Scott Lucett, eds. *NASM Essentials of Personal Fitness Training*. Burlington, MA: Jones & Bartlett Learning, 2014.

Hirotsu, Camila, Sergio Tufik, and Monica Levy Andersen. "Interactions between Sleep, Stress, and Metabolism: From Physiological to Pathological Conditions." *Sleep Science* 8, no. 3 (November 2015): 143–152. doi. org/10.1016
/j.slsci.2015.09.002.

Mayo Clinic. "Metabolism and Weight Loss: How You Burn Calories." Accessed on November, 14, 2020. MayoClinic.org/healthy-lifestyle/weight -loss/in-depth/metabolism/art-20046508.

Ratini, Melinda. "15 Things That Slow Your Metabolism." WebMD. Last updated September 23, 2020. WebMD.com/diet/obesity/ss/slideshow -slow-metabolism.

INDEX

ACKNOWLEDGMENTS

The production and completion of this book was a team effort. The shared knowledge of professionals led to the final product. A special thank-you to my editor, Rebecca Markley, for her feedback and writing expertise. Much credit goes to nutrition consultant Karen Frazier for her recipe contributions. Many thanks to all members of the Callisto Project team who each gave their time, energy, and effort to put together this amazing tool that can help so many people.

ABOUT THE AUTHOR

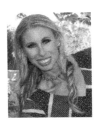 **Megan Johnson McCullough**, owner of Every BODY's Fit fitness studio in Oceanside, California, is an NASM Master Trainer, professional natural bodybuilder, fitness model, published author, and a candidate for a doctorate in health and human performance. Megan is also a Fitness Nutrition Specialist and Wellness coach. She holds an MA in physical education and health science and played college basketball. She currently seeks to help every BODY (hence the name of her studio) become the best version of themselves. She is happily married to her husband, Carl, and has two pugs named Steve Nash and Phil Jackson.